Nursing
and the law

Nursing
and the law

DAVID CARSON, LLB
Senior Lecturer in Law, University of Southampton

JONATHAN MONTGOMERY, BA, LLM
Lecturer in Law, University of Southampton

with
ELSA MONTGOMERY, BSc, RGN, RM

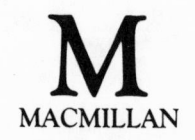

MACMILLAN

First published 1989

Published by
MACMILLAN EDUCATION LTD
Houndmills, Basingstoke, Hampshire RG21 2XS
and London
Companies and representatives
throughout the world

Printed in Great Britain by
Camelot Press,
Southampton

British Library Cataloguing in Publication Data
Carson, David
Nursing and the law
1. England. Medicine. Nursing. Law
I. Title   II. Montgomery, Jonathan   III. Montgomery, Elsa
344.204′414
ISBN 0–333–49572–1

Contents

Introduction

The past few years have seen many changes in nursing, nurse education and the management of the health service. The law that governs these areas has also been developing. The need for all nurses to appreciate and understand the role and potential contribution of the law has become obvious. This book hopes to meet that need, but it aims to go much further. Many nurses respond to the law with anxiety, because it is complex and uncertain, because it conjures up images of courts and civil or criminal liability, and for many other reasons. A better understanding of the law can relieve this anxiety and help both nurses and their patients.

The law provides a structure for nursing and has a role in the development of professional standards. While it is concerned with liability, it also protects and supports nursing values. We hope that this book will inform nurses about the law and demonstrate that it can be used to assist them and their patients. We have tried not to present the law as a series of rules of what may or, more commonly, may not be done. Instead, we have sought to explain the legal principles and show how they relate to the practical issues faced by nurses. In this way, nurses should be empowered rather than frightened by their knowledge of the law.

Our primary aim has been to make the law that is relevant to nursing practice accessible. We have deliberately avoided discussions of individual cases. These are too often confusing, and the details rapidly become outdated. A second motivation behind the decision arose out of the realisation that much of the literature on nursing and the law has been dominated by the concerns of other professionals and not geared to the needs of nurses. Most court cases have specifically concerned doctors: to recount them would have been little use in explaining the law that governs nursing. Furthermore, cases come to court when lawyers think there is an important issue, but what is important to lawyers is often peripheral to nursing practice. We have therefore asked ourselves what a nurse would want to know and sought to answer those questions. Keeping the lawyers' view under control has been a major task for the nursing part of the team: we have concentrated on the needs of nurses. Suggestions for further reading are provided for those who wish to explore the law in a more technical manner. Most of the material discussed in this book is also relevant to midwives and health visitors, but it would not have been possible to cover all aspects of the work of these professions adequately in the space available.

This book has been divided into three broad sections. The first section (Chapters 1 and 2) introduces the legal system and explains about the different kinds of law that apply to nurses. The second section (Chapters 3–6) refers to areas of law that apply generally to nurses in all specialties. The remaining section looks at particular groups of patients or clients. The law described is that applying in England and Wales. Although the laws of Scotland and Northern Ireland are often the same, there are sometimes important variations. There is considerable overlap between chapters, which is indicated by cross-references at the appropriate points. We hope that this will enable the book to be used both as an introduction and for reference.

We have agreed the final text of the book. However, primary responsibility for the initial drafts was shared between the two lawyers. Jonathan Montgomery wrote the first drafts of Chapters 4–6, 10 and 11, and David Carson those of Chapters 1–3 and 7–9. Elsa Montgomery has helped to set the agenda, provided examples from nursing practice and rewritten much of the book in order to make it comprehensible.

Both lawyers are working to develop, in conjunction with a School of Nursing, teaching materials on law and ethics relating to nursing. Therefore comments or suggestions about this book that might be incorporated into another edition and into that project will be gratefully received.

David Carson

Jonathan Montgomery

August 1989

CHAPTER 1

The law and nursing

Nursing courses have, for a long time, paid relatively little attention to the law. When it has been referred to it has often been seen as a series of constraints or threats: 'Do not do that or you will be legally liable.' The image has almost been of the courts waiting to catch someone out. Little attention has been paid to ways in which the law can help both nurses and their patients. This is not surprising. Attempts to use the law to gain greater resources for the NHS have failed. In marked contrast with the USA, it has been involved in few of the major changes in attitudes and services such as in community care and the introduction of the nursing process.

However, nursing has continued and is continuing to change. Nurses see themselves, much more frequently, as advocates for their patients, as being concerned with the whole person, with preventing ill health in its many forms. They are also gaining greater clinical independence and becoming more individually responsible. With these and other changes, nurses will become increasingly involved with the law and the courts. Instead of being 'victims' of the law, in the sense of 'falling-in' with whatever the law requires, they can and should be able to use the law constructively. Instead, for example, of just knowing that most patients must consent to treatment, nurses should be able to develop criteria of and tests for the existence of consent. In this way they can, at least to an extent, use the law to aid the goals, values and ethics that they hold dear.

This book aims to describe the law and indicate ways in which nurses can use it to their own and their patients' benefits. Naturally, however, it is not always easy. It is important to stress that the facts of each individual case that the nurse deals with will be critical.

Is the law properly followed in practice?

There is a difference between 'the law in books' and 'the law in practice'. The first refers to what is written down in statutes and textbooks or declared by judges. The second refers to what actually happens in daily life. They are not always the same. Sometimes this is because people deliberately break the law but, often, it will be because the law is misunderstood or is thought to be unfair or impractical. One example is the practice of obtaining relatives' consent to the treatment of unconscious or disordered patients. While this is a common practice, it gives no special legal authority for the treatment. Another example is defensive nursing where a practice is observed, such as rubbing the skin with alcohol before and after an injection, because it is traditional or it is thought that it would be negligent in law not to do so. As Chapter 3 explains, it is not negligent to stop a traditional nursing practice if the decision to do so would be supported by a body of responsible nurses.

The 'law in books' is about statutes and about the decisions of judges given in many cases. It is not about the individual facts of those cases. This rather obvious comment can be overlooked! Before declaring the law, judges must decide what the facts of each case are. The seeming ease with which judges declare the facts creates a false impression. Most trials are about discovering the facts rather than the law. The facts can be very complicated. The witnesses may sharply disagree. There may simply be very little hard evidence. And this can often occur in cases involving nurses. Patients will often be unable to notice or record what is happening; they could be under an anaesthetic, unconscious or severely mentally disordered. There may be few other witnesses to what happened, such as when nurses are working with individual patients or isolated from colleagues or other patients. It may be necessary to choose between the word of the patient and the word of a nurse. In court it is not just what happened that matters but what can be proved to have happened.

The courts will not become involved at all unless someone complains or otherwise initiates an investigation. Suppose a patient falls out of bed or a nurse divulges a patient's clinical records to members of the public. The law may, or may not, have been broken in each case, but if nobody reports the incident then nothing may happen. The law does not police itself, it relies upon someone starting proceedings. Failure to complain may be due to ignorance of the law, fear of people (including nurses) who still have some control over them, or for many other reasons including the cost of legal action. Certain practices can become so common or traditional that people begin to believe that they represent the law. For example, some believe it lawful to lock wards to prevent certain patients from wandering even though they are not lawfully detained patients. Another example is the belief that for there to be negligence there must have been a positive act, in other words, that an omission is not enough – that is false. Many more people could probably sue for medical negligence than actually do. Ignorance or misunderstanding of the law can lead to patients being unprotected. A particularly insidious example arises when ideas develop, from practice and experience, that, while nurses must not abuse patients, they are not obliged to protect patients by 'blowing the whistle' on their colleagues. As will be seen, nurses often do have such a duty.

Which is binding, law or ethics?

The law generally reflects current values and standards: supporting rather than challenging professional decisions on ethical issues. Judges usually appreciate that doctors and nurses are closely involved with the ethical issues and have to live with their decisions, and therefore defer to their greater experience and professionalism. However, there is much disagreement about ethical issues such as abortion, eugenics, heroic surgery and euthanasia. In such areas, decisions have to be made that will be contrary to some people's moral views. Some nurses may, from their personal ethical viewpoints, therefore disagree with the law. Only on some special occasions, such as participation in abortions, do they have a legal right to avoid involvement. On other occasions, for example responding to patients who have problems in expressing their sexuality, there are no special legal rights allowing nurses to avoid involvement just because it offends their personal ethics and values. Good employers minimise these occasions but, ultimately, nurses can be disciplined by their employer, by their professional body or taken to court. Belief in different or higher ethical standards is not a legal defence if the law is broken.

Must nurses obey all their employers' or superiors' instructions?

It has already been said that nurses may find themselves asked to do something that they believe to be unethical but which the law requires. If they fail to act, they may be legally liable for the consequences. They may be right, in the long term, just as we now recognise that many people who engaged in civil disobedience were right to disobey the law.

Nevertheless, the issues are very different when the instructions they are given are unlawful. It is no defence, in either criminal law or civil law, for a nurse to say that someone ordered her or him to do an unlawful act. If, for example, a doctor instructed a nurse to administer some medication that would, as the nurse realised, shorten the patient's life when there was no clinical justification for the medication (such as pain control), then the nurse could be as guilty as the doctor of both civil and criminal offences – if anyone complained. Superior orders are not a defence. If a nurse did not know that an instruction was improper or unlawful then she or he might be negligent for that ignorance (see Chapter 3). Ignorance of the law and/or good practice can cause harm rather than be a defence! Nurses should challenge instructions that they believe are improper, both for their own and their patients' good. Failure to question, to be assertive, could be negligent. However, the circumstances of each case, the facts, will be very important: for example, in an emergency, perhaps in surgery, where a doctor needs to make decisions fast and work fast. Exceptional circumstances often demand exceptional action and nurses following such a doctor's instructions, on the basis that he or she is the expert of the moment and questioning could cause harmful delay, would not be criticised for not challenging the doctor unless he or she had required something blatantly improper even in those circumstances.

Do nurses have contractual duties to their patients?

Nurses working in the NHS, including those working in general practices, do *not* have contracts with their patients. This is because our contract law requires that both parties must give something to the other. Nurses give services to patients but patients do not give anything in return. Praise and boxes of chocolates do not count. Nor do the patient's taxes count as they are 'given' to the government and only thereby, partly, used to pay for the NHS and nurses. So NHS patients cannot sue for breach of contract. The same would be true of most nurses working in private hospitals and nursing homes. They would have a contract with their employers, not with their patients. Nevertheless, those nurses who own nursing homes or are directly employed by a patient to nurse him or her, will have a contract with their patients. Those nurses employed and paid by others to nurse another person must be careful that their contractual duties to their employers do not conflict with their other legal and professional duties to the patient.

Having a contract enables both sides to enforce it. However, even broken contracts are relatively rarely enforced through the courts. Major reasons for making a contract are (a) to establish the relationship between the parties and (b) to stipulate the standards of performance and other expectations of the parties. Contracts are important in establishing the status of the parties. The person who is able to contract can pick and choose what he or she wants to happen. He or she is a consumer, is in charge and is responsible, rather than a supplicant asking and hoping for help. NHS patients do not have contracts and so cannot negotiate with doctors and nurses. They can be left to take what is available, to be dependent. Hence there is considerable interest in enabling patients to have contracts.

Making a contract presumes, and emphasises, the capacity and interest of the parties in making it. Hence contracts can reinforce the dignity of elderly, mentally-disordered and handicapped patients. However, treatment 'contracts' will rarely, in the public sector, be real contracts. They are useful ideas and encourage precision and agreement but very rarely indeed will they be legally enforceable. A patient may, for example, 'contract' to undertake a certain amount of exercise in return for a reward, but he or she cannot be required to undertake the exercise because of the 'contract'. The nurse is already obliged to provide the care and attention. The patient is not giving, in the legal sense, the nurse anything by acting in his or her own interests.

What kinds of law apply to nurses?

Nurses are, of course, citizens and subject to, and entitled to take advantage of, the law. They may, for example, use the law to protect themselves against their employers, perhaps for discrimination, unfair dismissal or not providing a safe place and system of work and adequately trained colleagues. They may use the law against patients who assault them or sue those who defame them. However, they may face difficulties if they use the law against their patients without consulting their employers first. The patient may not have been in control of him- or herself at the time of the incident. However, nurses are also subject to and involved with special laws on their own and their patients' behalf. Subsequent chapters will describe these laws. The most common legal action by patients is to bring a claim of negligence. This law, and how it can be used to devise a 'risk-taking' strategy, is discussed in Chapter 3. Other areas of civil law such as trespass and breaches of confidence are discussed, where they are most relevant, in relation to nurses' duties of confidence in Chapter 5.

Nurses can be, and have been, prosecuted for committing crimes. These range from assaults and theft of patients' property to manslaughter where a nurse's recklessness may have caused a patient's death. While patients sue using the civil law, it is normal for the police or Crown Prosecution Service to bring prosecutions under the criminal law. (Private prosecutions are possible, although unusual.) In criminal cases, the prosecution must prove their case 'beyond all reasonable doubt'. So some prosecutions are not begun because the prosecutor's advice is that there is insufficient evidence for a conviction. This can occur in cases where nurses are accused of abusing patients where there is insufficient supporting factual evidence. In civil cases and professional and employers' disciplinary procedures, the court or tribunal only has to be satisfied 'on a balance of probabilities', although they will take into account the seriousness of the consequences for the people involved, such as loss of employment. So the same nurse may not be prosecuted for abusing a patient, or may be found not guilty, but nevertheless have her or his dismissal from employment approved by an industrial tribunal, have his or her registration as a nurse withdrawn by the UK Central Council (UKCC) and be sued by the patient for assault or negligence.

So, to summarise, nurses are affected by several different kinds of law.

Criminal law

Nurses can be prosecuted for breaking the criminal law just like everyone else. Most prosecutions are begun by the Crown Prosecution Service. Patients can be prosecuted but nurses should consult their employers and the police before bringing a private prosecution. Nurses can be compensated, under the Criminal Injuries Compensation Scheme, without someone being found guilty by a court.

Contract law

Nurses can be disciplined by their employers under their contracts. The powers and procedures are discovered by studying the contract. Contracts can be re-negotiated. Unless directly employed by the patient nurses do not have a contract with their patients. Nurses can sue their employers for breach of contract.

Tort law

Patients have a range of rights that will be protected by the civil courts. These include the right not to be physically interfered with without consent or other legal authority, the right not to be negligently nursed and not to have confidential information distributed to other people. Nurses also have rights not to be injured through unsafe systems of work or inadequately trained colleagues.

Professional law

If a nurse is suspected of professional misconduct she or he can be investigated by one of the National Boards and the UKCC and have her or his registration removed.

Other procedures

There are other procedures that can involve nurses. Instead of going to the courts, a patient may complain to the ombudsman (the correct title is the Health Service Commissioner), who can hold a very detailed inquiry and make a public report; however, he or she does not investigate issues of clinical judgment.

How are nurses protected from invalid complaints?

Courts and other tribunals have procedures to decide which complaints are valid. In addition, nurses have extra legal and practical protections against patients' complaints. As explained in Chapter 7, some mentally disordered patients must get the High Court's permission before they can sue nurses. It is a disciplinary offence, in most nurses' contracts of employment, to make malicious allegations against colleagues. It is also defamation for someone publicly to say or write something factually false about another that leads to the latter's loss of reputation. It would not be defamatory for a nurse to tell a manager about her or his beliefs about another nurse, even if they proved to be false, provided that it is something the manager ought to be told and is told in good faith. This is called 'qualified privilege'.

CHAPTER 2

The legal structure of health care

Health care involves many professions. It is regulated in many ways including professional and personal standards, social standards and moral values. The law is also an important regulator. The legal regulation of nurses as a profession is discussed in Chapter 4. This chapter examines features of the law and legal system concerned with the organisation and delivery of health care that affect nursing. In particular it examines:

- the kinds of laws and rules that bind people working in the National Health Service;
- the legal powers and roles of the Secretary of State and health authorities;
- the extent to which health authorities can be obliged to provide services; and
- the main kinds of proceedings that can be taken against health authorities rather than individuals.

So this chapter is principally about legal structures and organis- ations' legal obligations. It does not give clear answers to questions about when the courts will interfere with health authorities' and clinicians' decisions because the law is still unclear and it would be improper to imply otherwise. The chapter ends with two practical sections giving advice about (a) the most efficient ways of finding and reading the law and (b) ways of analysing legal documents rather than relying upon others' interpretations. The points made here could also be used by nurses when they have to write documents that require careful use of language.

What kinds of law govern the provision of health care?

Many people claim 'It's the law!' in an argument or discussion. Often they are wrong. For example, many quote circulars or notices issued from the Department of Health as being law. They are not. Often they will be accurate and excellent summaries of the law, especially new laws, but they are not actually law. It is important both that nurses are not misled as to what is law and what is binding and that they do not mislead others.

Statute law and common law must be distinguished. Statute law is passed by Parliament. The common law is the collection of judges' decisions about the law on subjects where Parliament has not yet passed any statutes. So the structure of the National Health Service is laid down, in statutory form, principally in the National Health Service Act 1977. In contrast, the law of negligence is, with exceptions on a few detailed points, part of the common law. Major areas of our law are still governed by common law, including much contract law, the law of trespass and many criminal offences such as murder and manslaughter. Parliament can alter common law by passing a statute. The judges cannot alter or make statute law although they do have to interpret it and, in doing so, can give it meanings that may have the same effect as altering it.

What is statute law and how is it made?

'Statutes' is a general term covering Acts of Parliament and 'secondary legislation' (the latter also known as statutory instruments or regulations). An Act begins life as a Bill. It has to be debated and approved in both Houses of Parliament, the House of Commons and House of Lords. During its 'first reading' the title is simply formally read out by its proposer. During its 'second reading' the general principles are debated. Then it has a 'committee stage' where a committee of members consider it in detail. Each House appoints the members who are to serve on these important committees. Pressure groups, and those with strong views, can send briefing documents to Members of Parliament on the committee to try to get it changed. Then it has its 'report stage' or 'third reading' before the whole House when more changes can be made; for example, the government of the day can use its majority to alter anything that it does not approve of.

Passing statutes is a slow, complex and expensive process. In areas of law that change frequently, such as social security rates, a quicker and cheaper procedure is needed. So, many Acts include sections giving a Secretary of State the power to make regulations or statutory instruments. Instead of having to be debated several times by both Houses of Parliament, most statutory instruments are subject to a 'negative resolution'. That means that they will automatically become law, after a specified period, unless they are rejected by a vote – this would be very unusual since the government that introduces them will usually have a majority at each vote. Provided that these regulations are made in the proper way, and within the authority that the Act gave to the Secretary of State, then they are as much law as an Act.

However, there are several problems with statutes. They have to cover a wide range of people and events, so they often just list duties or minimum standards and rarely include statements of ideals or detail to cover all the many complex circumstances that can arise in real life. So some Acts have a section that requires a code to be drawn up, often after consultation with interested organisations. These codes have a special value in stating good practice and ideals. Once the code is drafted, the Secretary of State can officially recognise it. For example, the Mental Health Act 1983 refers to a code: however, the drafts have been attacked by various organisations and none has reached formal status at the time of writing. The legal status of each code has to be separately investigated. Often they have no legal force and their primary value is in enunciating agreed values. Sometimes, an Act will specify the Code's role and authority. For example, industrial tribunals can take into account a code on equal opportunities, but they do not have to. Section 2(5) of the Nurses, Midwives and Health Visitors Act 1979 empowers the UKCC to issue advice on standards of professional conduct for nurses and midwives. They have issued a code. However, while it is widely accepted as enunciating central rules and values in nursing, it is not directly binding on the courts. As discussed in Chapter 4, the code is used as a standard in disciplinary decisions but is not binding. Codes can, however, so closely represent standards that their lack of formal legal authority may be unimportant in practical terms.

Two Acts, affecting health and community care, give the Secretary of State special powers. Under section 13 of the National Health Service Act 1977, he or she can give health authorities a direction in writing, which they must obey. Under section 7 of the Local Authority Social Services Act 1970 local authorities must exercise their functions under any general guidance that the Secretary of State issues. These are separate and different from the circulars and notices issued by the Department of Health. Circulars and similar documents are not law and are not binding. While disregarding circulars may incur the Secretary of State's wrath, it will not be breaking the law.

An example may illustrate the different forms of legislation and non-legislation. The following legislation is concerned with the regulation of private hospitals, nursing homes and residential care homes. Some nurses work in them, while others will receive patients from or discharge patients to them and should be ▶

interested in how standards are enforced there. Some senior nurses will have the special responsibility of inspecting these hospitals and nursing homes and have powers to recommend closure!

- **Registered Homes Act 1984.** This *Act* governs the registration, inspection and supervision of private hospitals, nursing homes and residential care homes. It also covers withdrawing registration and rights to make representations and to appeal.
- **Residential Care Homes Regulations 1984** (S.I. 1984, No. 1345). These *regulations* specify the minimum standards that residential care homes must meet.
- **Nursing Homes and Mental Nursing Homes Regulations 1984** (S.I. 1984, No. 1578). These *regulations* specify the minimum standards that nursing homes must meet.
- **Registered Homes Tribunal Rules 1984** (S.I. 1984, No. 1346). These *rules* detail the constitution and procedures of the special tribunals that consider disputes about the registration of homes.
- **Home Life.** This is a *code* of practice for residential care.
- **Registration and inspection of nursing homes.** This is a handbook for health authorities.

The first of these *codes* above (Home Life) was produced by the Centre for Policy on Ageing, and the second by the National Association of Health Authorities. Government ministers had promised to implement codes once the legislation was passed. There is no reference to them in the Act. However, the Secretary of State announced, in the foreword, that Home Life was to be treated as if it was general *guidance* that he had issued under section 7 of the 1970 Act mentioned above. Thus it should be treated as binding. (A major problem in practice is that, even if binding on local authorities, it is not binding on the tribunals!)

- LAC(84)15, HC(84)21, LAC(86)6 and HC(86)5. These are *circulars* that have been issued in relation to the Act. They explain the law and describe a scheme for collecting information on home owners who lose their registration. In the second circular mentioned there is also a *direction* under section 13 of the 1977 Act that requires health authorities to search out unregistered nursing homes. (The abbreviations, LAC and HC, stand for Local Authority Circular and Health Circular.)

What is the common law?

Even when there was no parliament to pass statutes there were judges and laws. The judges declared the law through their decisions and some of these decisions were written down and preserved in law reports. Over time, consistent rules gradually evolved, which were sometimes amended and developed to meet new circumstances. The judges recognised the principle of precedent; if the law is interpreted in one way in a particular case then it should be interpreted in the same way in all other similar cases. Most, if not all, of us would regard this as only fair, just and sensible. And that is how it works in practice. The law of negligence, for example, is primarily common law. By studying judges' decisions on a range of negligence cases it becomes possible to predict what a judge will do in a particular case. However, it is not always easy. Each case will involve slightly different facts; the allegedly negligent nurse might have been a student rather than a charge nurse. The lawyers involved may wish to argue that those facts are sufficiently different from the previous cases, the precedent cases, to justify a different decision being made. The difference between being a student nurse and being a charge nurse could, quite easily, be significant in a negligence case, although insignificant in an assault or confidentiality case. So, if there are precedent cases (known by lawyers as 'authorities'), which a lawyer knows are unhelpful to the client, he or she will try to distinguish them by finding differences that justify having a different decision.

What is the role of the appeal courts?

It is always possible for judges to make mistakes. So there are rights to appeal to another, higher, court. Sometimes there can be several appeals, such as from the High Court to the Court of Appeal and on to the House of Lords. The last appeal court's decision will be the binding one. However, the appeal courts usually only consider questions of law. The High Court might, after hearing the witnesses and studying the evidence, decide that a nurse was negligent. The nurse may appeal to the Court of Appeal but the Court will not call and hear the witnesses again. They will study a transcript of the evidence. Appeal courts will certainly overrule a judge who got his or her law wrong, but they are reluctant to interfere with a judge or jury's finding of fact. They always say that the judge or jury observed the witnesses' demeanour and thus were able to assess how credible their evidence was. So lawyers look for a point of law to appeal on rather than relying upon a claim that the judge misunderstood the facts of the case.

Having appeal courts also allows the law to develop. If an interpretation of the law becomes outdated or is otherwise considered inappropriate, the appeal courts can review it and, by various devices such as distinguishing precedents, can change the law. The theory is that they are not making the law (that is for Parliament), but that they are declaring it. However, in practical terms, the significance of an appeal court's decision can be as important as a new statute; they can also have this effect upon statutes. The courts have to interpret statutes; however, on several occasions, they have interpreted them in ways that observers believe was contrary to what Parliament was trying to achieve.

What is the hierarchy of the courts?

The courts are organised into a hierarchy. Except at the highest levels they are also organised by the kinds of law that they deal with.

The House of Lords

This is the highest appeal court hearing civil and criminal cases. While also Lords they are all senior lawyers. They usually sit in courts of five and are addressed as 'My Lord'. They also serve on the Judicial Committee of the Privy Council, one of whose jobs is to hear appeals by doctors from the General Medical Council.

The Court of Appeal

This court hears many more appeals than the House of Lords. There is a criminal division that hears appeals against conviction and about sentence. They usually sit in courts of three and are addressed as 'My Lord', even when women, although they are not usually peers.

The High Court

This is divided into several divisions indicating particular kinds of law, such as the Family Division. The largest division is the Queen's Bench, which deals with negligence and many other subjects relevant to nurses. It also provides the judges for the senior Crown courts. Judges sit alone, except in criminal and defamation cases where there are juries, and they are addressed as 'My Lord' or 'My Lady'.

The Divisional Court

This court has a very special role. It hears applications for a 'case stated' (where a lower court states the facts of its case for the

Divisional Court to state the applicable law) and prerogative orders (discussed below).

The Crown court

This court deals with criminal cases. There are different levels of Crown court, with the more serious cases, such as murder, going to a more senior court. The High Court judges who sit in the senior courts and those in the Old Bailey in London are addressed as 'My Lord'. The other judges are addressed as 'Your Honour'. The judges sit with juries, who decide whether the defendant is guilty, while the judge tells them the law and imposes sentence.

County courts

This court deals with a wide range of civil cases, including disputes over children. The decision whether a case begins in a county court or the High Court largely depends upon the kind of law involved and the sum of money at stake. At the time of writing, major reforms have been proposed. The judge is addressed as 'Your Honour'. Within this court there is a Registrar who has a special role. He or she can decide 'small claims' under simplified procedures that are designed to enable people to bring their own cases without employing solicitors.

Magistrates' courts

This court is largely associated with criminal work but has many other roles such as in relation to domestic disputes, maintenance, child care and licensing. Its association with criminal work is said to discourage people from seeking its protection. This is one reason why family courts have been advocated. Most magistrates, also known as Justices of the Peace, are lay people advised by their clerk who has legal training. Some, in large urban areas, are stipendiary magistrates who are experienced, salaried, lawyers. They are all properly addressed as 'Your Worship'.

Other judicial bodies and tribunals

There are many other official judicial bodies and tribunals, for example the Mental Health Review Tribunals, which can discharge patients detained in a mental disorder hospital, and industrial tribunals, which consider claims of unfair dismissal from employment. Appeals, on points of law, from these and other tribunals can enter the court hierarchy, usually at the Divisional Court or Court of Appeal level and can, if permission is granted, go so far as the House of Lords. The Court of Protection, which manages the property of some mentally disordered people (see Chapter 8), is headed by a Master. It is not really a court but certain High Court judges can hear difficult cases in their court and their decisions can then be appealed.

What are prerogative orders?

Another role of the courts is to review the behaviour of central and local government, the decisions of public bodies and officials. This is generally described as the judicial review of administrative action. It is largely achieved by the prerogative orders. For example, an order of prohibition will prohibit a public body from doing something unlawful; an injunction can have the same effect. An order of 'habeas corpus' requires a person's detention to be justified. An order of 'mandamus' requires a public body to carry out its statutory duties. An order of 'certiorari' quashes an improper decision. And a 'declaration' declares the law by announcing whether the action being debated was lawful.

The orders are discretionary. Someone who has been detained in a hospital because of a suspected mental disorder, for example, is most unlikely to obtain an order of 'habeas corpus' because there will be paperwork indicating that the detention is likely to be legal even if the individual is not disordered. However, if a Mental Health Review Tribunal misunderstood the law, an order of 'certiorari' would quash the Tribunal's decision and indicate how to correct the decision. Nevertheless, it would still be for the Tribunal to apply the court's ruling to the particular case. These orders and procedures can be very important in the health services. For example, Mrs Gillick's litigation about contraceptive advice for children under 16 years was based on her application for a declaration that a Department of Health and Social Services circular stated the law incorrectly. While a declaration, unlike the other orders, does not actually have any legal effect in the particular case (in the sense of quashing a decision or requiring certain action), public authorities such as health authorities and social services departments, can usually be relied upon to change their behaviour to conform with them.

Can the courts tell the Secretary of State or health authorities what to do?

The National Health Service Act 1977 gives the Secretary of State a wide range of powers and some duties. For example, section 3(1) states that:

> It is the Secretary of State's duty to provide throughout England and Wales, to such an extent as he considers necessary to meet all reasonable requirements:
> (a) hospital accommodation;
> (b) other accommodation for the purpose of any service provided under this Act;

(c) medical, dental, nursing and ambulance services;
(d) such other facilities for the care of expectant and nursing mothers and young children as he considers are appropriate as part of the health service;
(e) such facilities for the prevention of illness, the care of persons suffering from illness and the after-care of persons who have suffered from illness as he considers are appropriate as part of the health service;
(f) such other services as are required for the diagnosis and treatment of illness.

The first thing to note is the distinction between a duty and a power. A duty is something that *must* be done, whereas a power is something that *may* be done. The second thing to note is the frequent inclusion of 'let out' words. In section 3, above, there are the phrases 'as he considers appropriate' and 'as he considers necessary'. Other examples include section 5(1) of the Chronically Sick and Disabled Persons Act 1970. This states that when local authorities provide public toilets they have a statutory duty to make provision for disabled people, but it is limited by the phrase 'in so far as it is in the circumstances both practicable and reasonable'. And section 2 of the same Act, which imposes a duty to provide various services, is limited by providing that the local authority must be satisfied that the services are necessary to meet the needs of the person. Unless they are so satisfied no duty will arise.

The third thing to look for is a section, usually near the end of the Act, that details what is to happen if there is a dispute about implementing the Act. Legislation about health and community care usually includes such a section giving the Secretary of State various powers to settle disputes and impose decisions. The national health legislation gives the duties and powers to the Secretary of State. It then authorises him or her to delegate them to Regional Health Authorities, and authorises them to delegate them to District Health Authorities. However, it also allows the Secretary of State to take back the powers and to impose Commissioners. Section 85 of the 1977 Act allows the Secretary of State to consider complaints about authorities and to declare them to be in default. If this happens, the members of that authority are dismissed and new members appointed. When such a section exists, the courts will conclude that Parliament meant that particular procedure to be used rather than the use of the courts' powers.

This explains why the courts are so rarely used to enforce rights to health care. The most likely reason for wanting to use the courts would be to try and get the government of the day to allocate more resources to health. The judges are wary of being pulled into political disputes and insist that others, such as health authorities, are better placed and skilled to decide how much resources should be allocated where, when and how. And governments will always be wary of committing themselves, through the language of statutes, to future expenditure that they cannot easily control. While rights may be written into legislation, often to create an impression that rights are being created, the broader laws and procedures about what the courts will enforce can prevent them from being enforceable.

Is there a legally enforceable right to treatment?

The courts do sometimes tell central government and other official bodies what to do or, more often, correct their decisions. They can also declare that subsidiary legislation, like regulations, is unlawful because it goes beyond the powers in the Act that established it. This is called acting 'ultra vires'.

There have been a few court cases on the right to treatment. For example, in *In Re Walker's application* (*The Times*, 26.11.87) the parents of a baby, which needed a heart operation, asked the Divisional Court to instruct their health authority to provide that operation. The Court, supported by the Court of Appeal, refused to issue that instruction. However, it does *not* follow that the courts would never do so. The particular facts of that case were critical. The operation was not immediately necessary to save the baby's life. Drugs and other forms of support were keeping the baby alive. Indeed, there were other children clinically assessed as having a greater need of an operation. If there had been a need for an immediate life-saving operation then the courts *might* have granted the order. Equally, it appeared that the hospital would then have performed the operation voluntarily. We have to write 'might' because it is a prediction based upon what the courts have said in cases with different circumstances and because the Court's language is ambiguous.

When asked to make a prerogative order, the courts will consider whether the official body or person in question is acting wholly unreasonably. This is *not* the same standard of unreasonable behaviour or decision-making that is used in the law of negligence, which is discussed in Chapter 3. The courts allow official bodies extensive discretion in how they interpret and carry out their duties. However, if it can be shown, for example, that they took into account improper considerations, or procedurally their decision was very improper, then the courts may issue an order. Thus, the decision not to provide an operation for the baby was, in the particular circumstances of the case, not wholly improper nor reached by an incorrect procedure. In another case, a woman was told that her health authority had insufficient resources to provide her with renal treatment to avert her premature death. Here the courts might have granted an order. This is a guess because, in the individual case, extra resources to provide the treatment were allocated when she indicated that she was going to the courts. The courts have made plain that they will only intervene in exceptional cases, for example where health authorities take into account improper matters, such as racial origin, or where their decision is thoroughly unreasonable. We have not had sufficiently clear judgments from the courts to be sure whether they would decide that it would be thoroughly unreasonable to refuse life-saving treatment just because of lack of resources. Equally, their response to decisions about providing scarce treatments to patients based upon their 'quality adjusted life years' can only be guessed at.

So the courts will rarely enforce a right to treatment. They will only get involved where the decision is clearly legally or procedurally wrong. This is not limited to cases where lives are at stake but such cases are probably likely to succeed. The courts have also indicated that they could use prerogative orders to review decisions such as detaining a patient under the Mental Health Act 1983 or refusing a woman fertility treatments because of her past life as a brothel keeper, which had no clinical relevance. There are other possible tactics.

- Patients could seek a declaration establishing their rights to treatment. These are discretionary. They do not require anyone to act although public bodies could, generally, be relied upon to respond. However, when they declare the law, the courts are likely to emphasise the degree of discretion the public bodies have in implementing them.
- Patients should consider whether they, already, have grounds for a case alleging negligence (discussed in Chapter 3). If a failure to provide treatment has produced loss, including financial loss, there *might* be a case.
- Patients could also try calculating the losses they will suffer if treatment continues to be delayed and put that cost against the cost of providing treatment now. That may, in itself, impress the authority into action but it could also, if the cost of delaying is greater than the cost of treating now, be used to suggest that the decision not to treat has been poorly made. However, this too would not be sufficient, in itself, to demonstrate negligence.

The courts have a limited role in enforcing a right to treatment. They are more used to compensating people after their treatment has gone wrong. However, patients can suffer to the same or a greater extent through not obtaining treatment. If greater attention was paid to the consequences of omissions then there could be a greater role for the courts.

How can one find out about the law?

There are many practical problems in finding out what the current law on a particular point is, even for lawyers with access to a good library. It is always important to check that statutes, for example, have not been amended and that the latest judicial comment upon a law has been noted. Nurses would be best advised to find a text book on the particular subject they are interested in. This should be about the broad subject and not just part of it; for example Professor Hoggett's book, *Mental Health Law*, looks at the whole subject and not just the Mental Health Act 1983 as many other books do. It is too easy for a book on a particular statute to ignore important parts of the common law or other statutes relevant to the topic. It should always be the latest edition because the law changes rapidly.

Loose-leaf encyclopedias can be very useful: two deserve a mention. Richard Jones' *Encyclopedia of Social Services Law and Practice* (published by Sweet & Maxwell) has a solid reputation and contains much relevant information for nurses, including the Mental Health Act 1983, Registered Homes Act 1984, all the statutes affecting the care of children and much of relevance to services for elderly people and people with physical disabilities. It comes in two volumes and several times a year new pages are issued, to supplement or to account for new developments. It too can be out of date but only by months rather than years. Most importantly, comments are added after each section of an Act discussing its meaning, purpose and any relevant case affecting it. It also includes summaries of some cases. There is also the *Encyclopedia of Health Services and Medical Law* edited by John Davies and Joe Jacob (published by Sweet & Maxwell).

If such encyclopedias are unavailable and a statute has to be consulted, it is wisest to consult them in *Halsbury's Statutes* (published by Butterworths). This is a collection of statutes by subject matter with editorial comments added, with special updating volumes that can be consulted about any changes since the original volume was printed. Some individuals and libraries have access to a computer data-base called *Lexis*. This contains all statutes, statutory instruments, cases from this country and the USA. Cases, including those not fully reported (as is quite common with cases concerning health services), are usually inserted within a couple of months. Statutes are amended whenever this takes place.

Many court decisions are published each year, but they are a small proportion of the total number. These reports are concerned with the law; cases that just involve a dispute about the facts would not be reported. Précis of some cases are reported in newspapers like *The Times*, *Guardian*, and *Independent*. Any judgment about the law can be used to support an argument in another court but, naturally, the higher the court quoted, the more authoritative will be the argument. The more official law reports are collected together in volumes, often by year. They are unlikely to be found in ordinary libraries. However several journals, such as the *Lancet* and the *Health Service Journal*, contain reports and discussions of cases of relevance to the readers of those journals.

How can the law be read and interpreted?

The law keeps changing. Nurses will need to keep up to date with changes affecting them, even though they have completed their training. Equally, they may be involved in drafting documents, such as care policies, where unambiguous and explicit writing is desirable. Frequently, people spread stories about what the law means, which others uncritically accept. This can be to several people's disadvantage, such as where nurses incorrectly advise patients about their rights. It is wise to refer back to the law and check its meaning. Several techniques can help in interpreting law.

Most legislation follows a pattern. Near the end of an Act, but at the beginning of regulations, there is often an interpretation section. Consult this early on to see which words and phrases have been given special meanings. Other common sections specify when the legislation is to come into force and which parts of the UK it applies to. Then it should be noted how sections are grouped around topics. Within a group of sections, the first section will, generally, state a broad rule with the other sections elaborating upon it. And, within a section, the first sub-section tends to state the general rule with the following sub-sections providing exceptions.

An example to illustrate how to interpret the law

Several techniques for interpreting law can be illustrated by examining the tests for receipt of the attendance allowance. This allowance is paid to long-term disabled people with more being paid to those who require attention or supervision during both day and night. The tests require that the individual is:

> so severely disabled, physically or mentally that, by day he requires from another person:
> (a) frequent attention throughout the day in connection with his bodily functions; or
> (b) continual supervision throughout the day in order to avoid substantial danger to himself or others; or
>
> . . . is so severely disabled physically or mentally that, at night:
> (a) he requires from another person prolonged or repeated attention in connection with his bodily functions; or

(b) in order to avoid substantial danger to himself or others, he requires another person to be awake for a prolonged period or at frequent intervals for the purpose of watching over him.

Do not ignore the short words
'The' implies one only in marked contrast to 'a'. 'And' and 'or' clearly have different meanings. However, the 'or' in 'physically or mentally' needs to be interpreted as 'and/or' to be sensible and 'the' before 'day' and 'night' should be interpreted as 'a' since particular days are not specified. 'All' should cover all cases unlike 'some'.

Look for causal connections, phrases or tests that are linked
Here the person must be 'so' disabled 'that he requires'. The 'continual supervision' must be 'to avoid substantial danger'. Examine these words closely and consider similar meanings. 'Requires', for example, implies 'needs' and 'depends upon'. It does not imply 'obtains' or 'gets' and yet many people have been refused the allowance because they were not getting sufficient attention or supervision. The word 'requires' should make it plain that it is not what people obtain that counts but what they need to obtain. Similarly 'to avoid' dangers should lead to investigators inquiring about all the accidents that have *not* happened, that is, 'have been avoided', and not just those that have occurred.

Consider the contrasting expressions
Here there are 'night' and 'day', 'attention' and 'supervision'. While these are vague words whose meanings slide into each other, for the purposes of this law they are distinctly separate ideas. The courts have said that 'night' and 'day' are ordinary words of the English language and must, therefore, be interpreted as ordinary English language users would use them. Unfortunately the court then gave them a most unusual meaning! It declared that 'night' was the period of darkness when the household closes down. Thus 'night' could begin at or after midnight. And if a household had a disabled child and disabled adult it could have two 'nights' each night with the first beginning when the child is told to go to sleep and the second when the adult's carer goes to bed.

Consider the alternative expressions that are used
Interestingly, while it is called the 'attendance' allowance that word is never used in the law; it is 'attention' or 'supervision'. Note the differences. If Parliament had meant to write 'attendance' rather than 'attention' then it could have done so. It didn't. So 'attendance' should be contrasted with 'attention' to ensure that only the meaning of the latter is used.

Note qualifying phrases
It is only attention or supervision 'from another person' and 'in connection with bodily functions'. Requirements for help from mechanical aids or guide dogs, for example, would not count.

Look for the qualifying words, adjectives and adverbs
These include words such as 'continual', 'repeated' and 'prolonged'. Contrast them with similar-meaning words so that their distinctive meaning becomes more obvious. For example, it is 'continual' and not 'constant' so that the attention does not have to continue all of the time. It is 'repeated' and not 'repeatedly', so it does not have to keep repeating.

Look for words that are absent
Check that missing words are not being treated as if there. Does, for example, the word 'every' appear before 'night' or 'day'? Many have read this legislation as if that word was there but, if Parliament had intended it to be there then they could have put it there. (The more likely story is that they too presumed it to be there!) So requirements for attention and supervision do not have to be met every day.

This example illustrates the advantages of studying the language of the law directly and not always relying upon stories about its meaning. Of course, the courts and tribunals do not always follow the rules. Still there are techniques available to be used.

CHAPTER 3

Standards of professional conduct

Nurses have considerable power in that patients depend upon them, directly and intimately, and their standards of professional conduct. If a nurse makes a mistake or drops below the proper level of care then harm may be caused to patients and to the public reputation of nursing.

There are four main ways in which the law works to maintain nursing standards.

1   The criminal law could be involved where the harm was deliberately or recklessly caused. It is, for example, manslaughter to cause a patient's death through recklessness or through intentionally committing an unlawful act that causes death.
2   The Nurses, Midwives and Health Visitors Act 1979 gives the UKCC the power to de-register nurses found guilty of professional misconduct (see Chapter 4).
3   Employers may, under the contracts that they have with each nurse, discipline and dismiss nurses (see Chapter 4).
4   The law of negligence allows patients to sue nurses and their employers for compensation, should they suffer loss through a nurse's carelessness.

This chapter will concentrate on the law of negligence, which is the most commonly used legal concept in maintaining standards. The concept is also frequently found in the other methods of enforcing standards, for example employers and professions may discipline staff and members for professional negligence and sometimes negligence constitutes a criminal offence.

To whom must nurses not be negligent?

In the course of their professional and private lives, nurses come into contact with many groups of people, other than patients, who could be affected by their actions. Professional standards emphasise nurses' duties to their patients. Does the law share this emphasis or do nurses have responsibilities to other groups as well?

A nurse will only be liable for negligence if she or he negligently causes loss to someone to whom she or he owed a *duty of care*. This is the first of the five tests, all of which must be satisfied, for negligence. It specifies the people who must not be injured by another's negligent behaviour. It specifies who is owed a duty; it does not refer to the content of that duty. Actors might offend their audience during a performance, but they will not be guilty of negligence as actors do not owe a duty of care not to offend their audience. Nurses clearly owe their patients a duty of care. That is easy. The more difficult questions include whether nurses owe duties of care to patients' relatives, to strangers they nurse, for example off-duty at the scene of an accident. It is for the judges to declare the rules about when duties exist.

A useful judicial statement of the duty of care is that you have a duty of care to all those people whom you can reasonably foresee might be harmed by your actions or inactions. This test provides some limits. While it is easy to think up fanciful or complicated ways in which we might injure other people ('If only I had stayed in bed . . .') the test requires common sense. If we foresee that our behaviour might harm someone we should stop and think whether we should continue with it. If our concern is fanciful or ridiculous, then the law says that we can ignore it without being liable. If it is reasonable to anticipate harm then, if we continue, the law requires that we accept the consequences. Nurses may, for example, be concerned about discharging an elderly man because his wife is not very fit and may be unable to look after him properly. Can those nurses reasonably foresee that, if they do not make a good decision about when to discharge and organise support in the home, that the patient or his wife, or both, may be injured? Is that reasonable? If 'yes' there would be a duty of care. (How well they act refers to the standard of care, discussed next, not the existence of a duty.) This reasonable foresight test is not the only one that the courts use. They take 'public policy' into account. They will not impose a duty of care if they conclude it would be manifestly unfair to do so or be contrary to a sense of morality.

The test applies to inactions. It is reasonably foreseeable that forgetting, or failing to check when there is cause to check, the correct dosage of a drug could cause harm. It also applies to giving advice. It is reasonably foreseeable that wrongly advising a patient that he or she would not be eligible for mobility allowance could cause harm. The duty is not restricted to patients or clients. It is reasonably foreseeable that failing to pass on critical information to colleagues could lead to harm to them. The duty is not limited to professional roles or work time. It is reasonably foreseeable that an off-duty nurse going to the aid of someone at the scene of an accident could cause harm if careless. So there could be a duty.

How can a nurse know whether she or he is being negligent?

If nurses owe so many duties of care to so many people and in so many different ways then, given that things sometimes go wrong, why are so few sued? If nurses' duties of care are not exclusively to their patients how are they to cope with conflicts of interests? To be liable for negligence it is not enough that there was a duty of care; there must also have been a breach of the *standard of care*. What these standards are is an issue for the profession concerned. A nurse is not negligent when she or he acts in the way that reasonably competent members of her or his profession would act. The courts listen to expert witnesses, from the profession concerned, who describe the appropriate standard of care.

This test does not require the highest standards. Expert witnesses should not be asked what they would have done, in the case being disputed, but what reasonably competent nurses would have done. While the courts reserve a discretion to intervene and declare that the profession's standards are too low, this power is rarely exercised. This test will not protect nurses involved in 'accidents' or misjudgments if reasonably competent nurses would not have made them. The test takes into account the circumstances occurring at the relevant time. So if there is a sudden rush of patients in casualty the test will be what a reasonably competent nurse faced with that emergency would do and not what she or he would do if given all the desirable time and equipment. However, it might be negligent to have failed to predict the emergency and take appropriate steps to minimise its impact.

A similar approach could be taken when there are insufficient staff or resources to provide what is regarded as good nursing or acceptable standards. Did the nurses respond in a reasonably competent manner given the problems of limited or reduced resources? Just as those responding to a roadside accident would be judged by the equipment they could reasonably be expected to have available and to use, so will the overstretched staff be judged by the reasonableness of their response to reduced resources. They cannot just give up. To fail to advise managers of the limited resources could be a breach of the standard of care.

The test requires nurses to practise up to a common standard but it does not require that nurses always do what the majority would do. An individual nurse may be rather unorthodox in the way that she or he practises. However, it does not follow, because the practice was unorthodox, that any losses were caused by negligence. Would a reasonably competent nurse have taken that decision? The courts recognise that without people doing things differently, challenging current procedures and practices, there would be no change and no progress. So there is no requirement to follow the majority. Indeed, to follow roles and procedures slavishly is to invite prob- lems as it implies: (a) a lack of thought about the individual case and whether a special different procedure is required; and (b) a failure to check whether those procedures are up-to-date and take account of modern thinking, research and practice. Indeed, it could be negligent not to be up-to-date with the literature on a subject.

The test takes qualifications and experience into account but also looks at the job being undertaken. Student nurses should be reason- ably competent in the tasks they are given to do. If they are not competent then their supervisor, the sister, charge nurse or other manager, may be seen as negligent in giving them work that they were not competent to undertake. The UKCC Code of Professional Conduct reflects the law when it encourages nurses to declare their incompetence in certain procedures rather than to try to undertake them. Nurses are entitled to support and training, and the failure to provide it might be someone else's negligence. Nurses are owed duties by other people, including their employers. (We are concentrating here on nurses' negligence.) An individual patient's losses may be the result of the negligence of several people. Each one would then be liable.

Can nurses rely upon the standards stated in the UKCC Code of Conduct?

The courts would, certainly, take the UKCC Code into account. However, it is written in rather general language. It was not meant to cover detailed individual examples. So a reading of the Code will rarely answer the question as to whether a nurse acted negligently or not. The Code is about principles and broad statements of standards. A distinction should be drawn between statements of (a) principles, and (b) standards. Principles, such as the rules of confidentiality, are rules that should always be obeyed unless an exception is available. Statements of principle can be stated relatively exactly. Standards, by comparison, should always be under review and changing – getting higher. They cannot be stated so exactly.

Should nurses practise defensively to avoid being sued?

Defensive nursing, like defensive medicine, involves providing the patient with tests, treatments and services designed more to protect the nurse or doctor from litigation or complaint than for the patient's needs. Certainly there will be liability if no reasonably competent nurse would have done, or not done, the procedures in question. However, provided there is support from a body (not necessarily the most or the best) of reasonably competent co-professionals, there is no need to be defensive. Indeed, undertaking further tests, for example, could expose the patient to more risks and extend his or her time in hospital. That could create liability if no reasonably competent member of the profession would have undertaken those tests! Unnecessary defensive procedures cost money, which could be better spent on treating other people with needs. For example, wiping the skin with alcohol before injecting has no advantage. If a responsible body of nurses were to decide that the money spent on such swabs could be better spent, they could decide to stop the practice without being negligent. Tradition, custom and practice can lead to poor nursing. The law does not require it!

One cause of defensive medicine and nursing is over-concentration upon the facts of previous cases where negligence has been proved. Previous cases can illustrate the application of the law but it can be dangerous to draw a general rule about the practice of nursing or medicine from the one case. For example, a court once condemned a nurse who failed to refer a patient presenting with a possible lump in a breast to a doctor according to agreed procedures. There could be cases where the nurse is as competent, as acknowledged by a procedure agreement, as a general practitioner in deciding whether such a patient should be referred to a consultant.

The correct approach involves isolating the particular facts and interpretation of the law upon which the case turned. Which core facts, if they had been different, would have led to a different finding? Then the facts of the case must be located in their history. Cases can take a very long time in getting to court. Standards may have changed considerably within that time. Courts judge on the standards that existed at the time of the incident. So it would be most unwise to generalise from facts based upon standards of, say, 10 years ago. The best approach is to keep considering whether a substantial body of professional opinion would support the proposed action.

Can nurses be sued if the negligent behaviour does not cause harm?

No, harm or loss must be experienced; and it must have been caused by the negligent act. The law requires that the breach of the standard of care causes the loss. These causation rules are legal rather than scientific rules. The particular negligent conduct does not have to be the sole or the main cause. It will be enough that it had an effect that was not insignificant or trivial. If there were several causes, then each cause can lead to liability although the total compensation awarded will not differ. The court works out who pays how much after it has decided that there is liability.

It may seem obvious that if there has been negligent conduct, and someone has suffered, then the one caused the other and someone will have to pay for it. However, this does not always follow! An important test is to ask whether the harm or loss would have occurred even if there had been no negligent conduct. For example, a child presents at casualty with injuries consequent upon falling out of a tree and he is cursorily examined and discharged. A few days later the boy has to be admitted for major emergency surgery because of injuries which were, negligently, not noticed at the initial examination. It looks as if the negligent examination caused the need for emergency surgery and resulting harm from delayed diagnosis. However, the harm to the boy might have resulted anyway; he might have suffered those injuries even if he had been correctly diagnosed and treated right from the start. The negligence did not make any difference. If this is proved to be the case, then the negligent conduct is said, in law, not to have caused the losses. There would be no liability in the law of negligence.

Nevertheless, these rules do not apply when disciplinary action is taken by the national boards of the UKCC or by employers. Employers and professional bodies can, and should, act on the bad conduct irrespective of whether it has caused harm.

Whose job is it to prove negligence?

The formal legal rule is that the plaintiff, the person who brings the case, must prove his or her case on the balance of probabilities. However, this rule should not be simplistically relied upon. It is for the judge to decide whether he or she is satisfied that the case is proved. Reports of judge's decisions will tend to show that the winning side's case was more believable. That is simply because the judge is explaining the reasons for his or her decision. If the parties to the case had thought that the evidence clearly favoured one side then the case would be unlikely to have gone to court. It would, like most cases, have been settled out of court.

The judges can be helped by using certain rules and inferences. *Res ipsa loquitur* means that the facts speak for themselves. There may be no direct evidence of, say, what a witness saw, but the facts might imply that there is only one proper conclusion to be drawn. For example, there may be no explanation as to how a patient actually came to be scalded in a bath but it must have had something to do with, the other evidence indicates, a nurse not supervising the patient properly. In such a case, the conclusion that the nurse was negligent might be drawn if there was no competing alternative explanation.

It will always be difficult for patients to prove exactly how the treatment they received while unconscious caused their injuries. However, since everything is within the control of the surgical team, an inference might be drawn that it was due to negligence. The plaintiff cannot prove it any further but the court will note that the surgical team is well-placed to disprove negligence. The formal rule is that patients must prove their allegations but it would be very unwise for any nurse to enter litigation simply defying the patient to demonstrate proof. It would be wise and helpful to try and isolate a non-negligent explanation for the losses.

What can patients be compensated for?

While the list of kinds of losses for which patients can be compensated is not closed, there are limits. Clearly patients will be compensated for physical harm. This will include actual extra expenses involved in remedying their injuries, including private treatment. It will include sums for pain and suffering, for loss of future earnings and loss of functions such as ability to see or walk. The amounts are related to previous awards, age, activity and other factors. There is compensation for recognised psychiatric disorders and shock. However, there is no compensation, for example, for simple sorrow or sadness.

The judges also decide, and it is a separate rule, whether the losses suffered should be regarded as too remote. It will rarely be relevant in medical or nursing accident cases but, if certain losses were of a kind that was not reasonably foreseeable, they will be declared too remote and not be recoverable. If nurses failed, for example, to use their powers to prevent a patient being treated for a mental illness from leaving hospital they could be liable for injuries to the patient (if all the tests of negligence were satisfied) but would not be liable to a jeweller for watches stolen by a patient who has no record of such behaviour. Again, the judges could rule that certain losses are not to be compensated for reasons of public policy. For example, the courts have refused to compensate people simply because they have been saddened by an incident, as opposed to suffering depression.

What happens if patients do not look after their own health?

It may seem that the only person not subject to duties is the patient. People who smoke or who do not look after their hearts should know that health problems are likely to result. Health visitors and others specialising in health education are not held to be negligent just because people do not heed their message. However, if a person, say with self-induced lung cancer, is negligently treated then he or she is as entitled as anyone else to seek compensation.

If a patient contributes to the happening of or the extent of his or her injuries there will be contributory negligence. In such a case, the court will assess the extent to which the patient has contributed to his or her injuries and reduce the compensation otherwise payable by that proportion. The patient will have to be negligent in the sense of not acting appropriately in his or her interests, and this will depend upon him or her having knowledge of what is appropriate. The patient who is led to believe that he or she must suffer in silence will not be contributorily negligent in having failed to insist upon a second opinion. The courts would take account of the age and illness or disorder of the patient.

Can the law of negligence be summarised?

Yes, the law of negligence can be summarised and a six-point checklist created. However, the ambiguity of the word 'negligence' should be noted. First, it can be used as a noun, as in this paragraph, to describe an area of law. Second, it can be used as an adjective or adverb qualifying the quality of conduct referred to in the specific incident.

1   Did the nurse have a duty of care? If 'yes' continue. If 'no' there can be no liability.
2   Was there a breach of the appropriate standard of care? If 'yes' continue. If 'no' there can be no liability.
3   Did the breach of the standard cause the losses? If 'yes' continue. If 'no' there can be no liability.
4   Are the losses of a kind recognised by the law? If 'yes' continue. If 'no' there can be no liability.
5   Were the losses too remote? If 'no' then there has been negligence. If 'yes' there can be no liability.
6   Did the patient contribute to the happening of or extent of his or her losses? If 'yes' there has been contributory negligence and the damages will be proportionately reduced.

An example of a negligence case is given below.

A woman was admitted to hospital having taken an overdose of drugs. Her stomach was pumped out and she was transferred to a mental illness ward where she was diagnosed as having a depressive illness with paranoid features. She had florid delusions about Christ, snakes and fires, and declared that she had to die. A registrar instructed that she was to be nursed on the ward but not subjected to constant observation. Some days later her husband, at the end of a visit, handed the charge nurse a box of matches saying that his wife had given them to him because she might otherwise use them on herself. This information was not put in the nursing notes. A few days later, although she seemed much improved, she went into the toilets, took out some other matches and set fire to her shirt. She was badly burned.

Her losses, physical injuries, were of a kind regularly compensated by the courts. They were not too remote, particularly given her preoccupation with death and fire! Clearly, both doctors and nurses owed duties of care to the patient. Did they breach the standard of care? Expert witnesses indicated that other reasonably competent psychiatrists would have given the same nursing instructions but that no reasonably competent nurse would have failed to record the incident about the box of matches. So the doctors did not, but the charge nurse did, break the standard of care. Did the nurse's breach cause the losses? The trial judge thought so but he was reversed upon appeal. Even if the charge nurse had recorded the incident the psychiatrist would not, the court agreed, have changed the nursing instructions. The incident would still have happened, the losses would still have been experienced. The nurse could be disciplined by his employers or the profession but was not liable in the law of negligence.

(*Gauntlett* v. *Northampton Health Authority*, 1985)

Does the law of negligence discourage risk-taking?

Reading about the law of negligence might frighten and discourage nurses from taking decisions, especially ones that are seen as being risky or being creative. However, the law of negligence can be turned round and used to guide sensible decision-making or risk-taking. It can become a valuable tool for analysing whether a proposed risk is sensible or not, whether it is likely to lead to legal action or not. If nurses can show that their actions were based on a sensible and thorough risk-taking procedure, they will rarely be found negligent. However, the procedure must be used when taking the decision and not just used to try to justify it after the event. While analysis after the event might show that the same decision would have been taken, and thus that the decision to risk did not cause the losses, disciplinary action could, and should, be taken for careless decision making.

The word 'risk' is vague. A distinction should be drawn between taking a risk and facing up to a dilemma. When taking a risk there is time to assess the possible outcomes and there is at least one option that does not involve the possibility of harm to someone. When facing up to a dilemma there are no solutions that are free of harms and there is a need to make a quick decision because delay is causing harm. If this distinction is accepted, it will be seen that many decisions taken by nurses would be better described as 'facing up to a dilemma' rather than 'taking a risk'. Health visitors involved in decisions about whether children should be placed under a 'place of safety' order are facing up to dilemmas rather than taking risks. If they do not remove the child, he or she may be further injured. If they do remove the child their relationship with the parents is damaged and the child may suffer through having an unsettled life. Higher standards must be expected from those who take risks, in this sense, than those who face up to dilemmas who are, effectively, dealing with an emergency. So if nurses describe their acts as risk-taking then they can expect the more demanding standards to be applied to them.

Nevertheless, what appears to be a risk could involve a dilemma. For example, the relative absence of activity and stimulation on a long-term ward could be seen as a harm to be weighed against the harms that might result from the patient being discharged. Either decision could involve harms; nurses must choose between them. Also, the recognition of the legal, civil, professional, employer's and social duties, could transform what appears to be a risk into the recognition of a dilemma requiring urgent action. A ward philosophy might emphasise the need for patients not to lose skills, to maintain their self-respect and to make decisions for themselves. Thus those staff will interpret failing to allow, or encourage, patients to take those decisions and do those things, as harmful.

When considering risks, pessimism can lead people to think exclusively of things that might go wrong. The benefits of risking often do not get as much attention although they are the justification for the proposed action. Also, when thoughts turn to possible harms, there is an understandable tendency to concentrate upon the worst possible things happening; for example, the patient who might be injured is considered as risking being killed. While this may appear to be playing safe, it really demonstrates a lack of attention to the

particular circumstances of each individual case and an unwilling-
ness, or inability, to assess the likelihood of each particular outcome.

It is also common to concentrate upon the patient or client and to
ignore the potential repercussions, good or bad, upon other people.
In deciding not to go for a place of safety order, to protect a child
whom it is feared might be being abused, there are certainly
possible good and bad consequences for the child. However, there
are also consequences for the parents, the quality of their relationship, their individual self-esteem, their rights, their attitudes towards
the child and towards their health visitors and the potential for future
collaboration for the child's benefit. These are all relevant, although
not equal, considerations.

Assessment of risks

Risks should be assessed using two measures: (a) the consequence,
the amount of good or harm that might result, and (b) the likelihood
of it resulting. Sometimes it is argued that other factors should be
considered separately. For example, some would argue that
surgery is more risky than medication; however, looked at more
closely the 'riskiness' is still measured by reference to the amount of
good or harm and how likely it is that that will happen. Both surgery
and medication can cause harm and good, and with different
likelihoods of causing good or harm depending upon the particular
treatment and patient. It is simply wrong to declare that surgery is
always more risky than medication.

Can a risk-taking strategy be summarised?

Risk or dilemma?
Analyse whether it is a risk or a dilemma. Consider whether any
duties, for example, legal, professional, ethical or social, urge you to
risk so that it is more akin to a dilemma.
List the benefits
List all the kinds of benefits that could accrue to (a) the patient or
client and (b) to others. This can include freeing a bed or other
resources to benefit others.
List kinds of harm
List all the kinds of harm that could occur to (a) the patient or client
and (b) to others.
What is likely?
Analyse the likelihood of each of the kinds of benefit and harm listed
above. Sometimes, it will be possible to use statistics of the prob-
ability of certain things happening, say of paralysis from a particular

operation; but, if not, an attempt should be made to think through, preferably with colleagues bound by the same rules of confidence to the patient or client, the most appropriate words to describe the likelihoods.

Consider the best action

Consider what action could reasonably be taken to increase the likelihood of the benefits being achieved and the harms avoided. Then take that action.

Obtain informed consent

Obtain the informed consents of the patient or client. The special legal meaning of 'informed consent' (see Chapter 5) is not intended here. It is, indeed, suggested that nurses could and should go beyond the minimum that the law requires. The fact that a patient or client wants to take the risk becomes a very important consideration for the benefits; the patient wants to take a risk and that is an expression of his or her legal right and self-esteem.

Get an informed second opinion

Consult and seek the support of relevant and informed colleagues for the proposed action. That you were not alone in your assessment of the risks, that colleagues and the client agreed, can only help. This is not to give those other people a 'veto' over the action but to encourage objectivity and to help prove that a careful decision was made. If anyone disagrees with the proposed action they should be required to specify their objections within the terms of this framework. Those points can then be considered and a reassessment of the risk made.

Assess whether the risk should be taken

Here a judgement must be made, which will often involve an assessment of values and imponderables. How is pain to be valued? However, following this procedure will demonstrate to others a clear attempt to be careful, objective and to consider all the issues.

Present the case

Present the decision as a decision to seek identified benefits in the light of identified harms occurring. If risks are taken in a hidden or embarrassed manner then that could invite inquiry. They should be seen as an integral part of the nursing function with an emphasis upon progress, dignity and rehabilitation for the patient.

Following a risk-taking procedure like this should help avoid legal and professional liability. It should also lead to more risks being taken because it emphasises the benefits of risking. Clearly, such an approach cannot be adopted for every decision but it is available for those more difficult occasions that professional judgement will identify.

An elderly woman has been in hospital because of an acute upper respiratory tract infection. The prognosis is that she is weak and cannot expect to live much longer. It is concluded that she is likely to live longer in hospital than at home where she would be alone and liable to fall and injure herself. She would like to go home. Should discharge be supported?

Is it a risk or a dilemma? Unless her decision can be invalidated by invoking the Mental Health Act 1983 or the National Assistance Acts (see Chapters 7 and 8) she has a legal right to leave hospital, nobody can detain her. There are important social and ethical values of enabling and respecting freedom of choice and privacy. Keeping the patient in hospital, when the hospital is not essential for treatment or diagnostic purposes, involves ignoring those rights and values and increases dependency. So, perhaps, it is a dilemma.

Discharging the patient might enable the patient to sustain relationships impeded by being a patient, prevent pets being destroyed, or enable someone else to have the hospital bed. It could lead to the patient catching a virus, falling, perhaps endangering others because she cooks by gas. She might not eat properly and starve. Some of these, in an individual case, may be probable or unlikely. The likelihood of at least some can be altered. A community nurse or neighbour might visit, a day-centre place might be organised. The cooker might be replaced, a smoke detector installed.

The patient has asked to go home. Does she still want to go home after she has been told the possible consequences? Do colleagues support the decision to allow her to go home, particularly those involved in providing community support? The decision can now be assessed. While this is only a superficial example it should be possible to consider very much more information in a particular case. So the decision may be taken to support this patient's desire and decision to go home to the surroundings she much prefers, in the knowledge that this might reduce her longevity and increase the chance of injuries, but after having acted to increase the benefits she can obtain from being at home and reducing the possibilities of harm to her and others.

CHAPTER 4

Nursing responsibility in context

The previous chapter considered the rules of law that govern the setting of standards for the nursing profession through the law of negligence. Those rules govern the conduct of individual nurses. They might seem to suggest that the law sees nurses as working in a vacuum, unconnected with fellow nurses, or with other health professionals such as doctors, anaesthetists and midwives. In fact, the law of negligence allows the context of nursing to be taken into account. Identifying the standard of care means asking how a responsible body of colleagues would have expected a nurse to act. Nevertheless, there are other ways in which the context in which nurses find themselves working is taken into account. This chapter is concerned with the principles governing the nurse's relationship with her colleagues.

Nurses must consider their responsibilities not only to those harmed by their acts or omissions, as discussed in the last chapter, but also to their colleagues in the nursing professions. This chapter covers three areas:

- the structure of professional accountability – the role of the UKCC and National Boards in relation to nursing discipline and the setting of standards for practice;
- the relationship between nurses and their managers – the effect of management policies on nursing responsibilities, the duties of managers to their employees and employees to their managers; and
- the position of nurses within the health care team – the position of junior nurses, responsible delegation, the significance of following instructions, and interprofessional relations.

Professional accountability

What are the UKCC and the National Boards?

The UK Central Council (UKCC) for Nursing, Midwifery and Health Visiting (to give it its full title) was set up by the Nurses, Midwives and Health Visitors Act 1979. This Act replaced the old system where the profession was placed in the hands of the General Nursing Council and several related bodies. The functions of the UKCC include:

- establishing and improving standards of training and professional conduct;
- determining the conditions of a person's being admitted to training and the kind and standard of training;
- providing advice on standards of professional conduct; and
- maintaining a register of qualified nurses, midwives and health visitors and regulating admission to and removal from the register.

The Council is made up of persons nominated by the four National Boards and by the Secretary of State. Most of the members will be nurses, midwives or health visitors, but those nominated by the Secretary of State need not be taken exclusively from these professions.

The National Boards are made up almost exclusively of members of these professions. A separate Board has been set up for each of England, Wales, Scotland and Northern Ireland. Each of them has two-thirds of its members elected by the professions, and one-third appointed by the Secretary of State for Health. The three professions (nurses, midwives and health visitors) each elect their own representatives. Nurses have the largest representation because they are the biggest group. The electoral system ensures a broad representation of views. Members hold their positions on both the National Boards and UKCC for five years.

The National Boards have responsibility for ensuring that the standards of training, set by the UKCC, are met. They arrange examinations prior to entry on the register and supervise the accreditation of courses. This involves investigation of courses offered by nursing schools when they are first set up and also periodically, ensuring that they have kept up with the current training needs of nurses and that they are being properly conducted. In addition to monitoring what is happening in nursing schools, the National Boards are concerned with promoting and developing new initiatives in nurse education. The training of the other two professions is similarly examined. Finally, the National Boards act as a filter to ensure that accusations of professional misconduct that have no foundation are rejected before reaching the UKCC itself for a full hearing. This is dealt with more fully below.

How are professional standards set out?

The main way in which the UKCC carries out the task of setting standards for the profession is by drawing up its *Code of Professional Conduct*. This Code is reviewed periodically. It was first issued in 1983, and the current edition dates from November 1984. It advises nurses of what is expected of them as professional practitioners. Its 14 clauses cover the priority to be given to the interests of patients/ clients, the nurse's responsibility to work with colleagues (both nurses and those from other professions), while making known to the appropriate authorities circumstances that jeopardise the interests of patients/clients and the expectation that nurses will not abuse their position for personal gain. Copies of the Code and other UKCC documents are available to nurses free of charge.

The UKCC has published further advice on two clauses of the Code: clause 9, which deals with confidentiality, and clause 14, which elaborates on the limits that the Code imposes on the use of professional qualifications for advertising commercial products. The obligation of confidence, as set out both in the general law and by the UKCC, is considered in Chapter 5, together with a discussion of the nurse's responsibility to respect the individuality of patients set out in clause 6. Other parts of the Code are not considered in detail in this book.

While the *Code of Professional Conduct* is the main tool that the UKCC uses to advise nurses on the standards expected of them, it is not the only one. When it appears to the Council that there are areas of nursing practice that give rise to confusion as to how professional responsibility should be exercised, it can issue guidance. Thus, in 1986, the UKCC published an Advisory Paper on the *Administration of Medicines*. This document advises nurses about their responsibilities in respect of the management of drugs and also encourages the development of appropriate local policies and guidelines. It is considered in detail in Chapter 6. The document *Exercising Accountability,* which gives advice on issues commonly raised, was issued in 1989.

How does the UKCC ensure that nurses meet the required standards?

No person is entitled to adopt the title 'nurse' unless entered on the register of qualified nurses. It is a criminal offence deliberately to deceive someone into believing that you are qualified when you are not on the register. The UKCC can therefore maintain standards by controlling the membership of the register. This can be achieved by refusing entry to persons who do not meet the required standards or by removing those who have shown themselves unable or unwilling to act in the way expected of them. In 1986, the UKCC introduced a system of periodic registration that requires nurses to renew their registration every three years to prevent it lapsing automatically. This is designed to ensure that only those who are still involved in nursing practice, and who can therefore be expected to have maintained their clinical expertise, have their names entered on the register. Previously, once initial registration had taken place, names were not removed except after a misconduct finding against the nurse, or her or his death.

Nurses can be removed from the register if they are found to be unfit to practise. This finding can be made on one of two grounds. First, that the nurse has been guilty of misconduct. This is defined as meaning 'conduct unworthy of a nurse'. Most cases will concern misconduct in relation to professional practice, such as failing to make proper notes after serious incidents have occurred. In such cases, an isolated incident will rarely suffice. Abuse of patients also constitutes a significant number of cases. 'Abuse' can include not only physical and sexual abuse but also theft of patients' property.

Not all incidents of misconduct arise in the immediate context of clinical practice. Nurses are expected to 'act, at all times, in such a manner as to justify public trust and confidence, to uphold the good standing and reputation of the profession' and 'to serve the interests of society' (from the introduction to the *Code of Professional Conduct*). Consequently, evidence of dishonesty and drug abuse is often taken as sufficient justification for removal from the register for misconduct. When a nurse is convicted of a criminal offence, the UKCC has to consider whether he or she has been guilty of professional misconduct. A conviction does not automatically mean that there has been 'misconduct': some offences will have no bearing at all on a nurse's professional work. What type of behaviour will be considered unworthy of a nurse will depend to some extent on the general climate of public opinion. In 1915, for example, a married midwife was 'struck off ' for cohabiting with a man who was not her husband because this was found to be unacceptable for a professional woman. Such a view would be unlikely to be taken today because public opinion no longer regards such behaviour as so outrageous.

The second ground on which a nurse may be removed from the register is that 'her fitness to practise is seriously impaired by reason of her physical or mental condition'. No blame can be attached to those who are removed from the register on this ground. Nevertheless, in order to protect the public it is necessary to ensure that all those permitted to practise as nurses are able to do so competently. Cases of this second type are dealt with by a separate procedure to misconduct cases because they raise different sorts of issues.

What happens when a nurse is accused of professional misconduct?

If an allegation is made to the UKCC or to one of the National Boards that a nurse is unfit to practise then it will be considered in accordance with a strict set of procedures. These are designed to protect nurses from malicious allegations, while ensuring that the public is safeguarded against incompetent practitioners. These procedures are set out in the Nurses, Midwives and Health Visitors (Professional Conduct) Rules 1987. Removal from the register can only take place after a full hearing of the case, at which the nurse's view of the matter will be considered. This hearing will take place before the Professional Conduct Committee of the UKCC, which is made up of at least three members of the full Council who are selected to ensure that the Committee has expertise in the fields in which the nurse concerned has been working. They will be assisted by a senior lawyer who advises them on points of law and procedure.

Many cases do not even reach the stage of a full hearing because they are rejected at a preliminary stage as being unfounded. Preliminary investigations are carried out by the relevant National Board. When allegations of misconduct are made against a nurse, the Board invites her or him to provide them with an explanation of the matter in writing. This covers both the nurse's account of the events concerned and her or his 'justification' of her or his actions. Many accusations are dismissed at this stage because the Board accepts the nurse's explanation, or believes that the allegations have no basis in fact. If they believe that there is enough evidence to require a full investigation then the case will be referred to the Professional Conduct Committee.

The nurse is entitled to be represented before the Committee by a friend, a lawyer or an officer of a professional organisation (such as the Royal College of Nursing) or trade union. The Committee will consider all the evidence. This includes allowing the witnesses to be cross-examined by the nurse or his or her representative. The nurse does not have to prove his or her innocence. Instead the allegations must be proved against her or him. If the evidence is insufficient, the Committee must declare that she or he is not guilty.

If, however, sufficient facts are proved, the Committee must decide whether they are serious enough to constitute misconduct. If they so conclude, they will then give the nurse a chance to explain his or her general circumstances before deciding what action to take. The Committee has three choices. It may take no formal action, but instead express its disapproval of what has happened and caution the nurse against repeating his or her behaviour. It may choose to postpone its decision in order to give the nurse a chance to improve his or her practice. Finally, it may remove the nurse's name from the register, either permanently or for a specified period.

What happens when a nurse is said to be unfit to practise due to ill health?

Like conduct cases, health cases go through a two-stage process. Sometimes it will appear that there are health problems in the course of investigations by the National Boards or the Professional Conduct Committee. If this happens, then those bodies will transfer the matter to the Health Committee of the UKCC, which comprises at least three members of a panel of twenty-five persons appointed from the Council itself. If it appears from the beginning that the matter concerns the health of the nurse, then the preliminary investigation of the matter will be carried out by a member of a panel of screeners especially appointed for the purpose. If the initial enquiries show that there is cause for concern, a full hearing before the Health Committee will take place. Procedural rules ensure that the nurse is protected against hasty and ill-informed decisions. As with conduct cases, the Committee will consider which of the range of possible actions is most appropriate.

How can a nurse challenge the decision of the UKCC?

If the decision goes against the nurse, the Act of 1979 gives nurses the right to appeal to the High Court. The Court will not decide for itself whether the facts of the case require the nurse to be removed from the register. It will, however, quash decisions that are made unfairly or unreasonably and, in cases of doubt, will order the UKCC to go through the procedure of hearing the case again. Decisions will be found to be made unfairly if the nurse has not been allowed to know all the evidence against him or her or to give a full explanation of the allegations. It is also unfair if a person already connected with the case, for example someone from the place where the nurse works, sits on the Committee. Sometimes the courts will decide that there may have been irregularities, but they are unsure whether there definitely were. In such cases, to ensure that the nurse has not been disadvantaged, they will order a rehearing by the Professional Conduct Committee.

Few decisions have been regarded as unreasonable but, in 1988, a court did so. The case concerned a nurse who had misread her patient's notes and administered the wrong drug. She reported the matter to the doctor supervising the clinic who assured her that no damage would be suffered by the patient (a child). The UKCC had 'struck her off' the register because they believed that the nurse should have informed her nurse manager of the mistake. The judge felt that no reasonable body concerned with the discipline of the profession could have reached this conclusion. There was no danger to the public because she had reported the incident to the doctor responsible for the patient. The UKCC had also failed to carry out its investigation fairly because the nurse was not given the chance to cross-examine the child's mother, nor to challenge accusations about her past conduct. The decision to remove the nurse from the register was therefore quashed.

If appeal to the courts does not result in the UKCC's decision being quashed, this does not necessarily mean that a nurse's career is over. The UKCC has the power to re-admit people to the register. A nurse may therefore apply to have her name put back on the register. This will usually occur only where she can show reasons to believe that she has reformed her ways so that misconduct will not recur. It is her job to prove her case for re-registration rather than the UKCC's to show that she remains unsuitable.

What duties do employers owe to nurses?

Employers' obligations can arise in three ways. Some will derive from express terms in the contracts under which nurses are employed. Some will not be written down, but will be implied from the circumstances, either because of the general law or because of the usual practice in hospitals. Finally, other obligations will be imposed by the law, for example duties in respect of health and safety at work and equal treatment. This section looks at some of the main duties but does not seek to cover all the aspects of employment law that affect nursing practice. Every contract will vary in detail and nurses should check their own to see what specific terms are included. The discussion here is concerned with general conditions that will be common to most nurses.

A safe workplace

Employers are required to check that the workplace is safe. This means taking responsibility for providing safe equipment and ensuring that hazards are removed promptly. It also means that employers will be liable if accidents occur because a nurse's colleagues are unsafe owing to incompetence. Consequently, many injuries that occur at work will give rise to the possibility of claims against employers, usually the health authority or the owners of the hospital or nursing home. In one case, a nurse injured her back when she tried to rescue a patient from a collapsing bed. The court found that the health authority was liable to pay her damages because they had failed in their duty to inspect the beds regularly to ensure that they were safe. In another a nurse recovered damages after slipping in a pool of water, which should have been cleaned up.

No discrimination on the basis of sex or marital status

A second set of obligations that are imposed on employers arise in the context of sex discrimination law. Employers are not entitled to discriminate on the basis of sex or marital status. Further provisions, both of English law and European law, require that equal pay be awarded to men and women for equivalent work. At the time of writing, the impact of this legislation on the nursing profession is still unclear. Although discrimination is assumed to be unlawful, it is possible for the employer to defend practices by showing that they are justified by the circumstances on non-discriminatory grounds. Cases of possible discrimination are probably best pursued with the assistance of trade unions and professional bodies.

Legal liability for the actions of employees

The third area of employers' duties concerns their legal liability for the actions of employees. Where injury has resulted from the negligence of an employee and which is related to their work, then the employers as well as the employee will be liable to pay damages to the victim. This is called *vicarious liability*. Unless they carry professional liability insurance, nurses will often have insufficient funds to pay any damages that are awarded against them, consequently it is more usual for patients to sue health authorities than the employees directly responsible for the accidents.

This has two important consequences for nurses. The first is that when a nurse is injured at work she will usually sue the hospital rather than the person whose individual actions led to the incident. The second is that, where patients are injured by the negligence of nurses, it is probable that they will not in fact sue the nurse herself. Instead, they will bring their action against the health authority, who may in turn sue the nurse to have her reimburse them for their losses. The court will then determine how much the nurse herself was to blame and will allocate her a share of the financial burden accordingly. In the NHS, it is unlikely that managers will ask nurses to reimburse damages unless they are insured against liability.

What duties do nurses owe their employers?

Contractual considerations

As the terms of contracts are a matter of agreement between the parties, the only limits to conditions that can be agreed are set by the general law of the land. Terms that require either the nurse or her employer to act illegally will be void and of no legal effect. So will terms that the courts consider to be contrary to public policy. Nurses should read their own contracts of employment to see what terms are expressly included. One of the obligations that will usually be put into nurses' contracts is that of confidentiality. This is in addition to duties of confidence that the nurse owes to her patients directly, and to her responsibilities to the profession. The details of this area of law and practice are considered in Chapter 5.

Common law considerations

In addition to the express terms of the contract, there are also obligations that bind all employees because of the general common law. The two most important ones for nurses are the duties of 'obedience' and 'good faith'. The latter requires nurses to refrain from activities that prejudice their employer's interests. This would include leaking sensitive information to the media, which would undermine the hospital's efficiency. An example might be revealing that a patient with AIDS or a famous person is being treated in the hospital. That is a breach of good faith that might lead to it becoming impossible to safeguard the patient's privacy.

The duty of obedience requires nurses to follow the instructions that their employers give them. There are however, limits to instructions that employers can legitimately give to their employees. Instructions that are either unreasonable or unlawful need not be obeyed. It is unreasonable to require nurses to jeopardise their own safety so, for example, a nurse who was instructed to lift a heavy patient without the appropriate equipment or assistance could refuse to do so. Nor can managers require nurses to act in a way contrary to their professional ethics. This is because nurses are employed to carry out professional duties and not to breach them. However, there is a difference between an instruction that clearly contradicts the professional code and cases where there is merely scope for differences of judgement. It is only the first type of case that justifies a refusal to follow instructions. This means that employers are entitled to expect that their policies on procedures are followed unless they are directly contradictory to nurses' professional obligations.

It is important to note that these are cases where the appeal is to some objective standard of reasonableness, not to the nurse's subjective views. Personal distaste for the actions required is insufficient. There is only one activity in which a nurse is entitled to refuse to participate on the ground that she personally disapproves of it. This is the Abortion Act 1967, which provides a 'conscientious objector' excuse, giving nurses a legal right to refuse to take part in abortions.

While it is clear that employers cannot require nurses to participate in unlawful acts, it is not always obvious what is lawful and what is not. In cases of doubt, nurses should seek the advice of their professional bodies. Sometimes issues can be clarified by recourse to the courts. In 1981, the Royal College of Nursing took legal action to determine the position of nurses who assisted in prostaglandin terminations. It was feared that this might be illegal under the terms of the 1967 Act because it was arguable that it was nurses rather than doctors (as specifically required by the Act) who performed abortions by this method. The House of Lords held that nurses would be acting lawfully provided that the procedure had been instigated on the instructions of a doctor. It follows that nurses cannot now refuse to assist in prostaglandin terminations on the basis that their role is unlawful.

What happens if contractual obligations are broken?

The usual remedies for breach of employment contracts are damages (compensation in the form of money) and disciplinary proceedings (only where the employee is in breach). The courts will not order employers to reinstate employees who have been sacked. A special statutory regime covers 'unfair dismissal'. This enables a nurse to take her employer to an industrial tribunal to claim damages. The definition of 'dismissal' includes 'constructive dismissal', where an employee has been treated in such a way as to force them to resign. Employees faced with possible unfair dismissal will usually be assisted by their trade union or professional body to fight their cases.

The structure of disciplinary proceedings will usually be set out in the nurse's contract of employment. Most commonly, this will be achieved by the incorporation into the contract of general rules, and in the case of NHS employees they will be those issued by the Whitley Council. In the private sector, each employer will produce their own disciplinary proceedings. A nurse may be immediately dismissed for very serious breaches of contractual duties without pay or notice. More commonly, even for cases of gross misconduct, either notice or pay in lieu will be given. The period of notice will usually be specified in the contract of employment, and is likely to be one month. For less serious matters a different framework applies. Initially an informal warning would be given. If the offence is repeated, this will be followed by formal warnings, verbally at first and, if necessary, again in writing. Should the nurse persist in her actions a final warning will be given. If this is ignored dismissal will ensue. For some offences of a more important nature, employers may 'leap-frog' the informal stage of this process.

When formal disciplinary steps are taken, the employee should be given notice that she or he is to be disciplined and has a right to call in a friend or trade union representative. A meeting will then be arranged at which the nurse will be informed of the allegations against her and allowed to explain herself. If the officer responsible for issuing the warning believes that it is necessary to investigate further in the light of this explanation, the meeting will be adjourned. Such further inquiries may, of course, result in the warning being dropped.

Where it is the employers who have failed to perform their obligations under the contract, the first means of remedy is to challenge their actions using the grievance procedures set up for that purpose. If this fails, the matter could then be taken to the courts in order to seek compensation. There, it will be necessary to show that the breach has led to damage quantifiable in terms of money. If this can be done, the employers will then be liable to reimburse employees for their losses.

Who is responsible for accidents that happen in the course of the work of a team of health care workers?

The final cluster of issues to be considered in this chapter arises because of the multi-disciplinary nature of modern health care. Unlike many areas of work, in health care many different professionals will be dealing with aspects of the same patient's care. This means that it is necessary to discuss the relationship between the different clinical responsibilities. Sometimes, it is possible to identify the individual whose mistake has caused an incident. If this is possible, then the only issue will be whether that mistake was negligent or in breach of professional or employment duties of that person. In other cases, it is necessary to determine who must accept responsibility for accidents that may have occurred because of a combination of minor mistakes, or through a failure of communication.

The courts are still developing techniques to deal with this type of situation. Two will be discussed here. The first is to hold the employer liable for any accidents. This is distinct from vicarious liability, where the employer pays for the negligence of the employee. Here, the courts have said that where it is unclear exactly who made mistakes, but all those who might have done so were employed by the hospital, then the hospital must pay. Thus, if a patient is injured because a monitor failed, it may not be clear whether the doctors and nurses used it incorrectly or whether the technicians responsible for it had failed to check it properly. The patient might not be sure who, if anyone, was negligent. Nevertheless, they might sue the hospital for failing to provide an efficient service.

The second technique is used where there is one person responsible for taking charge of the care at the time when the accident occurred. This has been used to hold surgeons responsible for errors made during operations. In one case, swabs were left inside a patient. It was unclear whether the surgeon was personally at fault because he had failed to check that nothing had been left inside or whether the mistake was made by a nurse who was counting the swabs. The court held that because the surgeon was 'in command' of the operation he had to accept responsibility. It is probable that this doctrine can only be applied in areas such as theatre nursing where there is a clear hierarchy of responsibility. On the wards, it will usually be inapplicable because, while the clinical responsibilities of nurses overlap with those of other professionals, they are not subordinate to them.

One particular difficulty facing nurses is raised by their relationship with these other professionals. Where it is clear that a person will have to accept responsibility if anything goes amiss, then it is probable that they should be entitled to control what occurs. Thus, in the course of an operation, nurses are expected to follow the instructions of the surgeon because it is the surgeon who will be found liable for accidental damage to the patient. However, this does not absolve the nurse of her own responsibility. The final section of this chapter therefore addresses the problems raised by the giving and receiving of instructions.

When must a nurse obey instructions she or he is given?

It will rarely be a sufficient excuse for a nurse's actions that she was only doing what she was told. As responsible professionals, nurses are accountable for their actions even when those actions involve following instructions. Conduct that is judged to be negligent by applying the tests explored in Chapter 3 does not cease to be negligent merely because someone else's advice was being followed. A responsible body of the nursing profession would not accept the advice of a hospital porter about lifting techniques. Therefore following the porter's advice would not protect the nurse from liability in negligence. The crucial question is whether a nurse's reliance on instructions would be supported by her colleagues. If not, then she will have been negligent.

There will certainly be some circumstances when it will be wholly responsible to accept the advice of other people. Where specialist expertise is involved, a responsible body of the profession, and therefore the law, would expect nurses to call upon those with the relevant clinical skills. Usually, a nurse who relies on the advice of the relevant practitioner will not be negligent even if the advice was in fact inappropriate and the specialist was found to be negligent. Nevertheless, nurses should still ensure that they take care to see that there are no obvious anomalies in the instructions they are given. The courts have suggested that it might be negligent to follow instructions that appear 'obviously incorrect and danger-ous' without challenging the relevant clinical specialist to check that they were in fact appropriate. It will normally be sufficient to satisfy the standard of care that the nurse has sought confirmation, it is not expected that he or she will question the clinical expertise of those from other professions if they stand by their original position. However, as liability depends on whether the nurse has been negligent, it is for the profession to determine when it will not be enough simply to check instructions. The circumstances in which they are given will be important. In emergencies, nurses will be more likely to be expected to obey without question because of the urgency.

The House of Lords has considered the extent of the duty to question instructions in connection with the responsibilities of junior doctors. There they suggested that there would be a duty not to follow such instructions, even after they had been confirmed, where they were 'manifestly wrong'. In that case, the clinical expertise of the junior was in the same clinical sphere as the senior. Where nurses are faced with instructions from members of other profes-sions based on expertise that they do not themselves possess, it is unlikely that they would be expected to refuse to follow instructions even here. Where they believe that the patient is at risk they could nevertheless choose to decline to follow the instructions. This would be an example of a case where employers could not accuse them of disobedience because such instructions would be directly contrary to the requirements of the obligation in the *Code of Conduct* to put the interests of patients first (see *Exercising Accountability* (1989), Section G).

The courts and the UKCC have accepted that responsible practitioners recognise their own limitations. The *Code of Conduct* requires nurses to: 'Acknowledge any limitations of competence and refuse in such cases to accept delegated functions without having first received instruction in regard to those functions and having been assessed as competent.'

The courts also recognise that one way of meeting the standard of care is to call for help when appropriate. Thus it will not be negligent if a nurse tries to provide the best care for the patient by confirming with superiors what course of action should be taken. Should the advice of the superiors turn out to be negligent, then liability lies upon the senior nurse not the junior. This is because the junior has done all that could be expected of her by a reasonable body of her peers. The converse of this principle is that nurses who are supervising or advising their juniors must take care to ensure that they do not give negligent advice. Nor should they delegate functions to nurses who are not competent to perform them unless a responsible body of nurses would also do so (see Chapter 3).

CHAPTER 5

The patient as an individual

Respect for the individuality of patients is a fundamental principle of nursing ethics. Clause 6 of the Code of Professional Conduct outlines one of the consequences of this principle where it says: 'Take account of the customs, values and spiritual beliefs of patients/ clients.' Nurses must be prepared to recognise that their patients are entitled to see things in ways that may seem strange and to have their choices respected even if they appear irrational.

The individuality of patients is protected when it is recognised that they are entitled to certain moral rights:

- the right to choose when to be left alone;
- the right to choose what happens to them;
- the right to know what is happening; and
- the right to their private affairs being kept private.

This chapter considers the extent to which these rights are protected by the law.

Do patients have a legal right to be left alone?

It is a basic rule of English law that no one has any right even to touch another person without their consent. So, theoretically, a nurse may not do anything to a patient unless they have first obtained the patient's agreement. The exceptions to this rule, which make the law less strict in practice, are set out below. If the nurse does proceed without consent they will be acting unlawfully and may be sued by their patient using an action called battery (sometimes known as trespass).

Unlike negligence cases, this legal action can be brought by the patient even if the care or treatment in question has not damaged them and even when it has been for their benefit. However, this will happen only rarely. Usually only nominal damages will be ordered if there has been no loss suffered.

It follows that the law relating to consent is very important for nurses. In order to be effective consent must satisfy several tests, set out by the law to ensure that the agreement is 'real' and not artificial.

1   The patient must be able to understand the nature of the choice they are making.
2   The consent must be 'free' or voluntary. Patients should not be pressurised into accepting a particular type of care, although a nurse may seek to persuade them to accept it. As one judge put it, a patient must consent to treatment not submit to it.
3   The patient must have been told in broad terms about the nature of the procedures in question. This does not require detailed information about the risks involved in the care or alternative methods of looking after the patient. Lack of detailed information will not invalidate the patient's consent. However, it may sometimes be negligent to withhold important information. This is discussed further below.
4   Consent must not be procured by deceit. Lying to the patient about the nature or effects of the care being offered will result in their consent being ineffective. This means that questions a patient asks about their treatment and care should be answered truthfully in a way the patient understands.

Are there any exceptions to the principle that consent is always needed?

The strictness of the consent rules is relaxed by the existence of exceptions. These exceptions are not mutually exclusive, and it might well be possible to justify performing a procedure without consent using more than one of them. The exceptions are listed below.

Exceptions to the principle of consent

Generally acceptable physical contact in ordinary daily life
There is a general exception to the need for consent that covers 'all physical contact which is generally acceptable in the ordinary conduct of daily life'. Thus those aspects of nursing care that involve only assisting the patient to do what he would normally do for himself will not, in law, require consent at all. Nevertheless, where the patient declines care even of this sort the refusal should be respected. This exception permits the nursing care of unconscious patients where the nurse is doing those things that they would normally do for themselves, but will rarely cover medical procedures.

In necessity
The principle of 'necessity' will sometimes justify actions where the patient is unable to consent to medical treatment or nursing care. This doctrine applies where the usual rules are superseded in order

to promote a more important value. The exact scope of the doctrine is unclear. There is no doubt that it permits life-saving treatment, provided that the patient has not previously expressed an objection to it. It probably extends to care given to prevent serious harm when it is not possible to get consent, either at all or in time to allow success. Nurses would be unwise to rely on this exception in less extreme cases.

Implied consent

It may be possible to imply consent in circumstances where it is thought that the patient would have consented had they had the chance, and so treat the case as if they had in fact done so. The most common situation where this doctrine might be used is where patients are unconscious, perhaps because of an accident or when undergoing surgery. In the latter situation, it may only become apparent that further surgery is required once the patient's body has been opened up, then the surgeon has to decide whether to perform the procedure immediately or wait for the patient to be able to consent and perform a second operation after explaining it to them. It is not clear whether this doctrine of implied consent exists in English law as no English court has yet had to deal with this area of law. If they do so, it is probable that they would apply the following tests, taken from the Canadian law, before they would accept that it was lawful to proceed without consent:

- the procedure must clearly be necessary for the patient's benefit;
- there must be no suggestion that the patient would object to it; and
- it must be unreasonable rather than just inconvenient to wait until the patient can consent if that will be possible in the future.

Summary

As can be seen, it will be very rare indeed that nursing care can be given against the wishes of a patient. There have been some cases where medical procedures that are life-saving have been found to be justified, but probably even here the basic rule that the patient's wishes should be respected applies.

What is the role of consent forms?

Consent can be given either expressly or by implication. In the case of medical treatment, it is usual to get the express agreement of the patient, often in writing on a consent form. In most circumstances, consent to nursing care will be given orally. Very often, nurses will not get express consent at all for nursing care, but will rely on implied consent. For example, if you explain to a patient that you wish to give them an intramuscular injection and they roll over, that implies that they agree to the procedure.

Providing the tests for the 'reality' of consent are satisfied, the form in which a consent is given does not matter. There is nothing magical about writing. Consent forms are used in respect of operations for two reasons. First, to make sure that consent is in fact given by recording it so that it is clear whether or not it has been obtained, and secondly to cover the doctor and health authority in case things go wrong. While it is unnecessary to get consent in writing, it is much easier to prove that consent has been given if a form has been used. If you think that something undesirable may occur in the course of a particular piece of nursing it is prudent to record the fact that you obtained the consent of the patient before going ahead.

The important thing, however, is the consent itself. The reality of the situation will prevail over the written evidence if there is a disagreement. Thus, if the patient does not understand the basic nature of the treatment, even if they have signed a form, the consent will be invalid. Equally, if the patient changes their mind this will override the written consent. With medical procedures, it is the doctor's responsibility to obtain the patient's consent. Nurses may feel that they should check that the patient is happy with his decision to accept treatment and that he understands the explanation given, but the law does not require them to do so. However, if a nurse has reason to think that the patient's consent might be invalid, then he or she should inform the relevant doctor in order to ensure that treatment is explained to the patient again. A failure to do so might be negligent (see Chapter 3).

Whose consent is required?

The need to consent is there to protect the individuality of the patient, and it is therefore the consent of the patient that is required. The only case where a third party's agreement is required by the law when the person to undergo treatment is capable of giving a valid consent himself is where the patient is a child and also a ward of court; then the permission of the court may be needed (see Chapter 10). Two cases that often give rise to confusion are abortion and sterilisation. The consent of the father of a fetus is not required before a woman undergoes a termination of pregnancy. The consent of a spouse is not required before a patient has a sterilisation operation performed, although it is often the practice for their consent to be sought.

Sometimes, however, a patient is not able to give consent. There are some special cases where another person may do so on their behalf:

- Parents will usually be able to give consent on behalf of their children (see Chapter 10).

- There are special procedures to deal with some cases where patients are unable to consent because of mental incapacity (see Chapter 7).
- Occasionally a patient may have arranged for someone to decide whether or not to consent on their behalf. Such a person may give a valid consent. Although the appointment of a proxy in this way need not be done formally, it would be wrong to assume that a relative can always consent on behalf of a patient. The usual practice by which the consent of the next of kin is obtained when a patient cannot him- or herself agree has no legal foundation unless a proxy arrangement has been made. However, it does demonstrate that you have not disregarded the patient's individuality, and will help ensure that the professional standards are met.

Must a nurse do whatever a patient asks even if it seems unethical?

Although a patient has a right that nothing is done to them without their agreement, this does not give them an absolute right to control what the nurse does. Sometimes a patient may request something that will be unlawful, such as help in ending their life or the infliction of serious physical harm; in such cases, the nurse may not lawfully comply. Two areas where the law restricts the choices open to patients are considered below. The first is choosing to die, the second is termination of pregnancy. Even where the patient's wishes are lawful, nurses are not obliged to comply with them. Whether they should is a matter of professional judgement and will be governed by the usual standards of professional conduct (see Chapters 3 and 4): Patients can therefore offer the nurses suggestions, with which they will usually wish to comply, but may not force a particular course of action upon them.

May patients choose to die?

Until 1961 it was a criminal offence to commit suicide. This meant that, until then, patients were not entitled to take steps to end their own lives. The Suicide Act 1961 abolished this rule. Under the old law, it had been the case that life-saving procedures, such as forced feeding, could be administered to objecting patients. This is no longer true. Where the patient is capable of taking the decision to refuse life-saving treatment rationally, his or her choice should be respected. If the patient cannot do this, a refusal of treatment should not be recognised. This leaves considerable scope for paternalism by health care professionals. A patient may be denied autonomy if those caring for him judge the refusal itself to be evidence of irrationality. The legal principle is that a patient is entitled to refuse life-saving treatment; the reality is that this right is poorly protected by the law.

Although a patient is entitled to refuse treatment, nurses may not assist them to die. English law does not permit 'active' euthanasia, where death is deliberately hastened. Such actions constitute a criminal offence under section 2 of the Suicide Act 1961. This offence is also committed if you assist or encourage someone to commit suicide. This does not prevent care that, although designed to relieve pain, also happens to shorten life. It is essentially a question of motive. To avoid committing an offence, any nurse who gives or assists in giving such care should first check that the care is designed to promote comfort not death, and second that it is the right and proper treatment for the patient's condition. This second requirement makes it largely a question of professional judgement.

The English courts have not yet had to deal with 'passive' euthanasia in relation to adults. One case relating to children, which will be discussed in Chapter 10, suggests that allowing a terminally ill person to die would be lawful providing there was no ulterior motive. The reasoning that supports this decision is suspect, and the law cannot be regarded as conclusively settled.

When is a woman entitled to terminate her pregnancy?

The second major area where the autonomy of patients to decide what happens to them is restricted by the law is that of abortion. Even when the woman concerned is satisfied that it is appropriate to terminate her pregnancy, further criteria have to be satisfied before the procedure may be lawfully carried out. The basic rule is that abortions are unlawful, but the Abortion Act 1967 permits them for some specific reasons. These differ according to the age of the fetus. The law divides the pregnancy into two parts. The line is drawn at the point at which the fetus becomes 'capable of being born alive'. This phrase refers to the possibility that the fetus could sustain its existence independently of the mother. The law presumes that this stage is reached by the 28th week of pregnancy. However, any fetus that could survive at an earlier age would be 'capable of being born alive'. Currently this is thought to mean that most fetuses of 24 weeks or more would be accepted by the law as being 'capable of being born alive'.

At all stages, a doctor is entitled to perform an abortion if it is necessary to save the life of the mother. Once the fetus has reached the stage of being 'capable of being born alive' this is the only ground that the law allows for a termination. However, in the first part of the pregnancy it would also be permissible to perform an abortion provided that two doctors have decided, in good faith, that one of the following two reasons for doing so exist:

- that the risks that the continuation of the pregnancy presents to the woman's life or to her health (physical or mental), or that of any existing children of her family, are greater than those that are involved in terminating it; or
- that there is a substantial risk that the child would be seriously handicapped owing to physical or mental abnormality.

Thus the control that mothers have over their bodies is limited by the constraints that the law imposes in order to protect fetuses. It must be said, however, that there is wide variation in the way in which the Abortion Act is interpreted by doctors. Some take the view that any pregnancy can be terminated because continuing a pregnancy is always more risky than ending it. Others allow abortions only in extreme cases. This means that abortions are very much easier to get in some places than in others.

How much are patients entitled to know about their treatment?

The principles of autonomy and individuality would indicate that patients should be entitled to information about their condition. However, English law does not give patients the right to know everything about their treatment. Although judges have suggested that when the patient has requested specific information they should be given it, negligence must be proved before a court will intervene in cases where the complaint is that insufficient information has been given to them. This means that everything depends on the standards that the profession sets for itself (see Chapter 3). Usually, cases of this kind concern doctors rather than nurses, and for them it is the standards of the medical profession that are relevant. The courts have suggested that the judges might set standards of disclosure themselves in some contexts, but have so far failed to do so.

The judges have, however, given some guidance to health professionals about disclosing information. They expect them to start from the assumption that patients would be told everything, but have recognised that there may be good reasons for withholding information. The main ones are:

- That the information is obvious and the patient can be expected to know it already: in such cases you can wait for the patient to ask.
- That it is such a minor piece of information, for example a minor side-effect that is very unlikely to materialise and that it is not worth mentioning.

- That the effect of knowing it would be to prevent the patient taking rational decisions about their treatment.
- That the patient's health would be damaged if they knew.

They have also suggested that patients should be told about alternative courses of treatment and care and about risks that might be particularly significant to them. However, if legal action is taken against the nurse for withholding information, it will turn on whether she has failed to live up to the standards set by her profession rather than whether these judicial recommendations have been followed.

Patients have no general right to see their notes, although professionals may decide to let them if they wish. There are three exceptions to this position. First, if a legal action is started, then the courts will order that the relevant notes be produced. Second, the Data Protection Act 1984 gives people a right to see information that is kept about them on computer. However, there are special rules dealing with health information, which means information that health professionals (including registered nurses) either hold or originally recorded or caused to be recorded. In respect of such information, access may be refused to a patient if: (a) it might cause 'serious harm' to their physical or mental health; or (b) it would enable the patient to identify someone else as the subject or source of the information contained in the records (except where the only such person is a health professional who has been involved in the patient's care). Where the information is sought from someone who is not a health professional it may not be revealed before a professional has been consulted to see if the exceptions apply. The appropriate person will usually be the doctor with responsibility for the patient's clinical care. These rules only apply to records kept on computer.

Finally, the Access to Medical Reports Act 1988 provides patients with a right to see medical reports made by doctors in respect of employment and insurance matters. The Act also gives them the right to forbid the release of the report, or to add explanatory comments if they feel it is appropriate. The Act does not apply to medical *records*, only to *reports*. It deals with employment and insurance reports because there are particularly strong arguments for patient access in those contexts and because these are areas where the spectre of HIV/AIDS has given rise to difficulties.

What information about a patient must nurses keep confidential?

Nurses acquire information about their patients from many sources, and it is likely to come to them subject to an obligation not to reveal it. The obligation applies to everything discovered about a patient that is not public knowledge. Subject to strictly defined exceptions, any revelation of such confidential information will be a breach, as will carelessly enabling an unauthorised person to discover it. Thus a nurse who allowed her sister to read the case notes of patients on her ward was found guilty of professional misconduct by the UKCC Professional Conduct Committee. The fact that she did not live in the area, was unlikely to meet the patients concerned, and was trusted by the nurse to keep the information secret was no excuse (*Nursing Times*, 26.3.86).

To decide whether information is confidential, consider the things you know about a particular patient, then ask yourself:
1 Does everybody know them? Public information cannot be confidential.
2 Do you only know it because you are a nurse?
3 Did the patient trust you to keep it secret?
When you answer yes to either of the final two questions you must keep the information confidential.

What action could be taken against nurses who reveal confidential information?

Three types of action might be taken against a nurse who breaches confidence. The UKCC might be asked to consider whether she had been guilty of professional misconduct, the nurse's employer might dismiss her for breach of her contract with them and the patient might sue her in the courts. For the UKCC, it is sufficient to justify action that a nurse has betrayed her duty of confidentiality under Clause 9 of the Code of Professional Conduct:

Respect confidential information obtained in the course of professional practice and refrain from disclosing such information without the consent of the patient/client, or a person entitled to act on his or her behalf, except where disclosure is required by law or by the order of a court or is necessary in the public interest.

The UKCC has given further guidance as to the meaning of this obligation in their advisory paper *Confidentiality: an elaboration of clause 9* (1987). Some of their advice is discussed below. The action that might be taken against nurses by the UKCC for breaching the obligation is discussed in Chapter 4.

A nurse's contract of employment will contain a requirement that all confidences are kept secret. Breach of this condition will not give rise to a legal action by the patient, but would provide a ground for dismissal by the employer, even if no patient had been harmed.

In the law courts, although the obligation itself is no less strict, it is unlikely that a nurse will be penalised unless the patient has suffered damage as a result of the disclosure. If this happens, the nurse may have breached the duty of care that she owes to her patients – she may be negligent. This will happen if confidential information is negligently disclosed when it is reasonably foresee-able that the patient will suffer from the disclosure. In one case, a doctor was held liable in negligence for revealing to his patient's husband that he considered her to be paranoid. He had not told her because it might have damaged her mental state and their relation-ship. Although the exact circumstances in which the husband revealed this information were not reasonably foreseeable, that it would cause harm was: the doctor was therefore negligent.

A nurse who has exercised reasonable care (see Chapter 3) to keep information secret will not be liable for negligence. This includes not only ensuring that she does not actively reveal infor-mation, but also that no opportunity is given for unauthorised persons to acquire it. Thus the RCN advises nurses working in occupational health to keep records secure under lock and key. Equally, the reasonably careful nurse should avoid giving confidential infor-mation over the telephone where 'it is difficult, if not impossible, to identify callers', and where conversations may be overheard (*Guidelines on Confidentiality in Nursing*, RCN, 1980).

Are there any exceptions to the obligation of confidence?

The obligation of confidence is subject to several exceptions, but nurses must assume that information should be kept secret unless it is clear that one of them applies. They are discussed in the UKCC's advisory paper. The exceptions are:
1 where the patient consents, or
2 where someone needs to know information to care for the patient's health, or
3 where the law requires or permits disclosure, or
4 where the public interest outweighs the obligations of secrecy.

Consent of the patient

As the obligation of confidence is owed to the patient, it is logical that he can release the nurse from it. Wherever possible therefore, the patient's advice should be sought at an early stage as to who they desire to know what about their health or circumstances. Relatives have no right to information unless the patient has agreed to the disclosure. If the patient is incapable of consenting to the disclosure because of his or her physical or mental condition the RCN advises that the nurse should seek the consent of the next-of-kin. This practice has never been considered by the courts, but would probably be sufficient to satisfy the nurse's duty of care. It is best to assume that the patient is capable of consenting, as it will be rare for a patient not to understand the meaning of their right to secrecy.

The need to know

Many health professionals need to collect information about the patient to carry out their tasks. One doctor has estimated that up to 100 people had access to his patients' records for either therapeutic or administrative purposes. If the obligation of confidence were absolute, record keeping would itself be a breach. This would clearly hinder, not enhance, the patients' care. Thus it is not a breach of confidence to disclose information to those who 'need to know' the information to perform their health-care tasks. Information relating to the patient's medical condition can therefore be legitimately passed on to other health care professionals. Some social history, but not necessarily all details of the patient's life, will be relevant. However, nurses should not reveal information unrelated to the patient's health.

Disclosure required by law

Health professionals are sometimes required by the law to reveal confidential information to certain public authorities. Responsibility for taking steps to report information falls upon medical practitioners rather than nurses, but nurses may lawfully be asked to provide information in connection with such matters. Examples of areas where disclosure is required by law include:

- Information that might lead to the identification of those involved in motor accidents must be given to the police. Gunshot wounds should be reported.
- Abortions and serious drug addictions are centrally recorded, and, in order to ensure that these records are as accurate as possible, they must be reported to the Home Office.
- Reporting of the 'notifiable diseases' (for example, cholera, plague, typhus and smallpox) is required (see Chapter 11).

Other statutory provisions do exist, but there is no general obligation to assist the police with their inquiries by revealing confidential information. Should a nurse wish to reveal any, she might be justified on the basis that it was in the public interest to do so (see below) but the police can only force disclosure in court. A nurse who is asked to give information should check with the health authority's legal department or with a professional body such as the RCN before revealing it.

The duty of confidence does not override the duty to give evidence in court. A nurse may not withhold confidential information if a judge orders that it be revealed in court. Confidences will usually be respected wherever possible. Nurses should ask the judge whether it is necessary to reveal the information, and do so only on the judge's instructions. A nurse who refused to obey such instructions would be in contempt of court.

Sometimes the law permits disclosure without demanding it. Under the NHS (Venereal Diseases) Regulations 1974 limited breaches of confidence are authorised, so that the disease may be prevented from spreading, or to facilitate the treatment of sufferers. Provided the information is given only to medical practitioners or those 'employed under' their 'direction', these disclosures will be lawful. These regulations do not allow a nurse to be forced to reveal information.

Public interest

This final exception provides the most difficulty. It is potentially the broadest, and the least defined. The RCN suggests that serious threats to individuals other than the patient, including the nurse and other colleagues will be sufficient to justify disclosure (*Guidelines on Confidentiality in Nursing* RCN 1980, para. 4.2). It will also be permissible to reveal information where there is 'a serious threat to the community'. The UKCC cites child abuse and drug trafficking as examples (*Confidentiality: An elaboration of clause 9* UKCC 1987, para. B.6). Breaches under this exception should be limited to the immediate needs of the situation.

Nurses working in occupational health face particular difficulties. The RCN has produced detailed guidance that provides further information in a document called *Practical aspects of confidentiality relating to the health of employees* (1986). Briefly, the nurse's duty to keep secret information relating to the patient takes precedence over her obligations to the employer. The employer's interest is not the same as that of the public, and information may not be revealed without the patient's consent. It may be advisable to get the employee's (that is, the patient's) agreement to the nurse's general opinions being conveyed to the employer at an early stage, perhaps before any consultation takes place. This would reduce the risk of misunderstandings. Detailed information about the patient should not normally be revealed.

CHAPTER 6

The administration
of drugs

This chapter considers the special problems that arise in connection with the administration of medicines. These are often dealt
with by the law as specific applications of the principles discussed
in Chapters 3–5. Where this is so, only a brief summary will be given
here and the relevant chapter will be indicated. There are also
special rules designed to reduce the risks of accidents concerning
drugs and to facilitate victims of accidents getting compensation.
Much of this law affects manufacturers, pharmacists and doctors
rather than nurses. The areas discussed here are those that affect
nursing practice.

Where is the law on drugs to be found?

The most important legal provisions that directly affect nurses are
set out in the Misuse of Drugs Regulations 1985, made under the
Misuse of Drugs Act 1971. They deal with prescriptions, specifying
the information that they should include, and with record keeping.
They are supplemented by the Medicines (Prescription Only)
Orders which govern medicines that may only be given on prescription but are not classified as 'controlled drugs' (see below).
The UKCC has produced an advisory paper *Administration of
Medicines* (1986), which offers guidance to nurses about their
professional responsibilities and discusses the impact of the
legislation. It is also common for managers to lay down local codes of
practice by which nurses will be bound under their contracts of
employment (see Chapter 4). These may impose greater restrictions than the law, for example, in respect of safe-keeping, the
witnessing of administration and disposal. Nurses should check
their local policies to see how they diverge from the general
provisions that are discussed here.

How are drugs classified?

Within the statutory framework governing the supply and control of drugs, there are three sets of classifications. The first derives from the Medicines Act 1968 and divides drugs into three categories: (a) prescription-only medicines; (b) non-prescription medicines available only through a pharmacist; and (c) general list medicines, which need not be obtained through a pharmacy. The Medicines Act contains provisions relating to the storage and sale of medicines and detailed rules governing the work of pharmacists. It also sets up a Committee on Safety of Medicines, which issues licences for drug trials and administers a reporting scheme to collate information gathered by doctors about side-effects of particular medicines. In this way, the Act seeks to protect the interests of both existing and future patients.

The second set of classifications is found in the Misuse of Drugs Act 1971. This Act is largely concerned with drug abuse, but contains important provisions dealing with the use of drugs in health care. It draws up a class of 'controlled drugs', which is subdivided into Classes A, B and C. Drugs are placed into these divisions according to how dangerous they are. Controlled drugs are identified in the Second Schedule of the 1971 Act by name. The Department of Health can alter the schedule and periodically drugs are added to the list, moved from one class to another or, less commonly, removed from it. Hospital authorities should have a current list, which can be consulted in cases of doubt. All controlled drugs come into the category of prescription-only medicines for the purposes of the Medicines Act.

The third set of classifications is used in the Misuse of Drugs Regulations 1985. These Regulations divide 'controlled drugs' into five categories. These are identified by the schedule of the Regulations into which they are placed. The controls placed upon drugs differ according to their schedule. Examples are used here to illustrate the scheme; however, the full lists are much longer. Schedule 1 contains the drugs that are most severely restricted; it includes non-medical drugs such as cannabis, raw opium and lysergide. Schedule 2 drugs include dextromoramide, dextropropoxyphene, diamorphine, dihydrocodeine, fentanyl, methadone, morphine and pethidine. Among the drugs in Schedule 3 is pentazocine; whereas diazepam, lorazepam, nitrazepam and temazepam can all be found in Schedule 4.

There are special rules requiring controlled drugs to be kept secure in locked rooms or cabinets. Employers will usually have devised local schemes to ensure that these requirements are met. The responsibility for drawing up schemes will rarely fall on nurses working in the NHS or in large hospitals, and their primary duty will be to follow the local protocols. In smaller private nursing homes, it may be nurses who are required to draw up such policies.

Who may administer prescription-only drugs?

Section 58 of the Medicines Act 1968 makes it an offence for any person to administer a prescription-only medicine to another unless they are acting in accordance with the directions of a doctor or dentist. The specific rules setting out the form that these directions must take in order to be valid are discussed below. Some exemptions exist, such as for midwives and occupational health nurses for certain drugs, but most nurses are bound by the general rule. Especially restrictive rules apply in relation to drug addicts. Only doctors specifically licensed to do so by the Home Office may prescribe drugs to addicts. The law does not provide further guidance as to who may administer medicines, but the UKCC has considered the matter, and most employers have drawn up special procedures to deal with the administration of drugs.

The UKCC believes that RGNs, RMNs and RSCNs should be competent to administer medicines without assistance. Enrolled nurses would not be expected to be able to do so without having been given further training. They note that the *Code of Professional Conduct* requires nurses to acknowledge their limitations and would expect nurses to refuse to administer drugs without assistance where they felt that patients might be put at risk.

Most commonly, managers adopt policies that are more restrictive than the legal and professional requirements. They will often require the administration of medicines to be witnessed and checked whatever the status of the nurses involved. Most local policies also require regular checks to be made of stocks of restricted drugs that are kept on wards. Such requirements are more extensive than those of the law. Employers are entitled to expect that their policies are followed and failure to do so might lead to disciplinary action (see Chapter 4).

What form must a valid prescription take?

Under the Misuse of Drugs Regulations 1985 and the Medicines (Prescription Only) Orders, prescriptions must be dated, written in ink or some other indelible material and must be signed by the prescribing practitioner. Certain information must be included. This covers the name and address of the person to be treated (in hospitals this is satisfied by writing the prescription on the patient's case sheet) and the dosage to be taken. In the case of controlled drugs this information must be personally handwritten by the prescriber. In addition, where controlled drugs from Schedules 1, 2 and 3 are to be given, the dosage must be written in both words and figures in order to avoid mistakes and alterations going undetected. In some circumstances, pharmacists may amend prescriptions, for example to avoid dangerous interactions between medicines. This should be done only after consultation with the prescribing doctor and, provided the alterations are signed by the pharmacist, the validity of the prescription will not be affected.

What duties do nurses have to check that prescriptions are correct?

Unless the prescription complies with the requirements set out by the Act, it will not be valid. If it is invalid, medicines dispensed under it will be given unlawfully. This will usually concern pharmacists. Nevertheless, where drugs are taken from a supply kept on the ward, it is important that nurses check that the correct procedures have been followed. Supplying a prescription-only drug without a valid prescription is a criminal offence. Where nurses have doubts about the validity of a prescription, they should not administer the medicine without contacting the prescribing doctor to have it properly written. Where that doctor cannot be contacted, the UKCC advises that nurses should seek advice from another doctor, a pharmacist or the senior nurse to whom they are responsible.

Responsibility for ensuring that the correct dosage of a drug is given falls primarily on the doctor prescribing it. However, in some circumstances, the nurse may share some of the responsibility. These are cases where she has acted negligently (see Chapter 3). For example, a reasonable nurse is expected to check the dosages written up for a patient, and if there is anything that seems unusual about the dosage she ought to raise it with a doctor. Nurses are expected to be familiar with the usual range of dosages of drugs that they commonly administer and to check those of which they are unsure (for example, with the British National Formulary). The nurse's responsibility is to raise the alarm, not to ensure that the dosage is correct. A nurse will not be negligent just because the dosage given was incorrect, but she might be if the error was such that any responsible nurse would have realised that something was wrong and she did nothing about checking it (see Chapter 4).

If the prescription is questioned and the doctor confirms it then the nurse has probably done her duty so far as the law is concerned, even if the doctor is mistaken. It may be that professional responsibility demands that nurses require the doctors to administer the medicine themselves where they believe that it is not in their patient's interest to do so (see Exercising Accountability (1989), Section G). In such cases, their obligation as employees to carry out their responsibilities in accordance with the hierarchy of authority set up by the employers will be outweighed by their professional duty to safeguard the interests of the patients/clients. In such cases, a nurse would be entitled to refuse to administer the medicine (see Chapter 4).

The most common problems concern dosages that seem very much larger than is usual, or where drugs seem to have been prescribed for the wrong patient. The courts have sometimes found nurses to have been negligent in cases where they have taken no steps to verify the prescriptions. They have not penalised them for the mistakes made in the process of writing up the drugs, as that is the responsibility of the prescriber. Two other things should be performed by nurses as part of their duties of care when giving medicines to their patients. The first is to check that the drugs are not beyond their expiry date. The second is to report any effects to the prescribing doctor. This is particularly important where there are unexpected or adverse reactions. Where side-effects of the medicine are observed, the doctor should inform the Committee on Safety of Medicines. This enables information on drugs to be collated, although it is generally thought that doctors often fail to report to the Committee. In addition to reporting these effects to the appropriate doctor, the nurse should record them in the notes.

What special rules govern record keeping in respect of drugs?

Records relating to controlled drugs from Schedules 1 and 2 must be kept in a special register. It must take the form of a bound book so as to ensure that records are not lost and to make it more difficult to alter entries. The quantities of controlled drugs added to the store, or supplied from it must be entered. Records should be indelibly made, in ink or some other suitable material and must be kept for at least two years. The regulations say that entries should be made on the same day as the supply of the drugs that they record. If this is not practicable, the register must be completed on the next day without fail. Separate parts of the register must be kept for some particularly dangerous classes of drugs. Local policies should provide guidance. They may well use the most restrictive provisions as their model.

Most employers will give guidance as to the frequency with which the stock of drugs kept on wards or in nursing homes should be checked against the records. This is a matter of local policy rather than legal requirement, although failure to check at all might well be negligent, both on the part of the nurse and also on the part of the management.

In what circumstances will the victims of defective drugs be able to get compensation for their injuries?

Patients may suffer from adverse reactions to drugs. The general law of negligence may give them a right to compensation (see Chapter 3). A doctor who prescribes a drug when he or she ought to have known that it was incompatible with medication that the patient was already receiving might be negligent in doing so. Manufacturers might be negligent in the course of making the drug if they do not take reasonable precautions to detect defects. Nurses who administer drugs incompetently might fail to satisfy the standard of care expected of them. Often, however, accidents involving drugs are not the result of any individual's fault. To deal with these cases, there are also special rules, which give rise to 'product liability'. These rules make producers liable for their products, and are important in respect of injuries caused by medicines.

The Consumer Protection Act 1987 gives those injured by defective goods (including drugs) a right to sue the producer of those goods. Under the Act the meaning of 'producer' is extended to include not only manufacturers, but also those who market or import goods into this country. The most important thing for nurses is that the Act is drafted in such a way so as to allow the victim to sue the person who supplied them with the drugs, unless that supplier identifies the producer. The definition of supplier here would include nurses, doctors and pharmacists. The right to sue the supplier can only be exercised by victims when they cannot identify the producers themselves and when they approach the supplier within a reasonable period after the damage was caused.

The existence of this legislation makes it especially important that proper records are kept, so that nurses can absolve themselves of responsibility by being able to identify the drugs that were administered to any patient. The Department of Health has issued a notice, HN(88)3 'Procurement Product Liability', to assist health authorities deal with their obligations here.

It should not be thought that these product liability provisions make it easy for the victims of drug accidents to sue. Experience has shown that it is very difficult to prove that injuries were caused by the drugs. Furthermore, the Act allows the manufacturers a defence if they can show that the state of scientific expertise was such that they could not have been expected to be aware of the defect. As many side-effects can only be discovered once drugs are in use, this defence may lead to the failure of many claims. These difficulties have led to the government setting up a special scheme to provide compensation for victims injured by vaccines. This is found in the Vaccine Damage Payments Act 1979. It created tribunals to ensure that victims get compensation inexpensively and quickly. It does not apply to all vaccines and does not offer large sums of money, but many who would not have been compensated at all under the general law of product liability have received money through this scheme.

CHAPTER 7

People with a mental disorder

People with mental disorders present nurses with special problems – legal and moral as well as clinical. Major issues of civil liberties are involved. Some patients with mental disorders can be detained and treated against their wishes. Other patients may comply with the suggestions of doctors, social workers and nurses only through fear of being detained. Many, whether in hospital or not, lose the right to manage their own property and income. Most of the special legal powers and procedures are given to doctors to exercise, but nurses working with people with mental disorders are in a particularly powerful position to protect and enhance the rights and dignity of their patients – or to abuse them. This chapter describes:

- the legal role and powers of nurses involved in detaining mentally disordered patients
- nurses' legal powers to restrain mentally disordered patients and to be involved in treating them against their will
- when patients can be prosecuted for their crimes
- the law relating to patients' sexual expression and potential liability of nurses.

The laws concerning the property of people with mental disorders are described in Chapter 8. Most people with mental illnesses and mental handicaps live in the community; however, this chapter will use the word 'patients' irrespective of where the person lives and whether obtaining health services. This is also the approach of the Mental Health Acts.

Is there a special law for people with mental disorders?

The general law, as described in Chapters 2–5, applies to everyone until specific exceptions are made. People with mental disorders have full civil and legal rights until a specific law decides otherwise. So there is, for example, no legal right to intrude into a person's private house, to restrain, to lock a patient in a ward, to treat without consent or to divulge confidential information just because the person has a mental disorder. Nurses must be able to provide a legal justification for treating a patient with a mental disorder differently from other patients. This chapter explains ways in which differential treatment can be justified. While courts may be sympathetic to their problems, nurses should never assume that judges will support them just because they acted competently, in good faith or in the patient's best interests. One person's view of good faith and best interests may be another's patronising interference with basic civil liberties. The courts will, within limits, protect patients' rights to be individual and to make unwise decisions. However, nurses would have to justify any failure to become involved with a patient who is acting dangerously or unwisely with his body or money. For example, some disordered patients wish to exercise their legal right to commit suicide, but any nurse who owes a duty of care to such patients might be legally liable for failing to act to prevent that suicide.

So patients with mental disorders can pose some exceptional problems for nurses but, generally, the law supports nursing goals. Mentally disordered people often experience multiple disadvantages, such as poverty and isolation. The law's values and goals of respect for patients' individuality, the requirement of their consent and the presumption of patients' competence to make decisions, complement nursing goals and philosophies. So the law can be seen as providing a foundation for advocacy for patients rather than being a hindrance.

What is 'mental disorder' in the law?

There are several different legal definitions of kinds of mental disorder. They differ from clinical definitions. For example, the definitions in Section 1 of the Mental Health Act 1983 govern detention, compulsory treatment (discussed in this chapter) and the involvement of the Court of Protection (discussed in the next chapter). However, those definitions do not apply when considering criminal liability, capacity to make a contract or the validity of a marriage. The correct definition must be used on each occasion. So, in this book, the definition must be discussed each time. While clinical services are divided between mental handicaps and mental illnesses that is not a particularly important legal distinction. In this chapter, 'mental disorder' covers both mental illness and mental handicap unless the context specifies otherwise.

Section 1 of the Mental Health Act 1983 provides the definition of 'mental disorder' that governs most of the issues to be discussed shortly. (Scotland and Northern Ireland have their own legislation, which differs in some details.) 'Mental disorder' is the collective term. There are five subdivisions, which are important because patients cannot be detained for more than 28 days unless they come within one of the first four categories in the box below.

Definition of 'mental disorder'

For each category, each part of the definition, in the following, must be satisfied.

Mental illness

This expression is not defined in the Act.

Psychopathic disorder

This requires: (a) a disorder or disability of mind, which (b) is persistent, and which (c) causes (d) abnormally aggressive or seriously irresponsible conduct.

Mental impairment

This requires: (a) an arrested or incomplete development of mind, which (b) includes significant impairment of intelligence and (c) significant impairment of social functioning, and which (d) is associated with abnormally aggressive or seriously irresponsible conduct.

Severe mental impairment

This requires: (a) an arrested or incomplete development of mind, which (b) includes severe impairment of intelligence and (c) severe impairment of social functioning, and which (d) is associated with abnormally aggressive or seriously irresponsible conduct.

Any other disorder or disability of mind

This catch-all category will include all those people with mental handicaps not covered by the 'impairment' definitions, at least some people with personality disorders and adults experiencing brain damage. However, people may not be regarded, in law, as mentally disordered 'by reason only of' promiscuity, immoral behaviour, sexual deviance or dependence upon drugs or alcohol.

Quoting the International Classification of Diseases should assist in determining the meaning of 'mental illness'. While with 'psychopathic disorder', the disorder must actually cause the conduct, this is not necessary with either form of 'mental impairment', where it need only be associated. Most people with mental handicaps will come within the 'any other disorder or disability' category as they are not associated with aggressive or irresponsible behaviour. While drug addiction and other behaviour are not to be treated as signs of disorder on their own, the phrase 'by reason only of' would permit them to be used as evidence of disorder provided they were cited with another disorder such as depression.

Can the sections under which patients are detained be summarised?

The principal sections of the Mental Health Act 1983 that allow patients to be detained are summarised in the box below. Subsequent parts of the chapter elucidate the major implications for nurses and their patients.

Summary of powers to detain patients

RMO = responsible medical officer; ASW = approved social worker; NR = nearest relative.

Treatment order (section 3)

This order lasts six months, on first renewal for another six months, and on subsequent renewals for a year at a time. It applies to the four specified disorders and is made by the NR, or by an ASW if the NR does not object, on the recommendations of two doctors.

Hospital order (section 37)

This order lasts six months, on first renewal for another six months, and on subsequent renewals for a year at a time. It applies to the four specified disorders and is made by a Crown or magistrates' court on the recommendations of two doctors.

Assessment order (section 2)

This order lasts for up to 28 days. It applies to all five forms of disorder. It is made by an ASW or the NR on the recommendations of two doctors.

Emergency order (section 4)

This order lasts for up to 72 hours. It applies to all forms of disorder. It is made by an ASW or NR on the recommendation of one doctor.

▶

Voluntary inpatients (section 5(2))

This order lasts for up to 72 hours. It applies to all forms of disorder and to voluntary inpatients who seek to leave the hospital. It can be made by the RMO or one other doctor nominated by the RMO.

Nurses' power to detain (section 5(4))

This order lasts for up to six hours. It applies to all forms of disorder and voluntary inpatients who seek to leave hospital. It can be made by any nurse on the appropriate part of the professional register (parts 3 and 5).

Can patients be detained for prolonged periods?

Different sections of the Mental Health Act authorise the detention of different categories of patient for different purposes for different lengths of time. The 'treatment order' enables a patient to be detained for six months, renewed for another six months and then for a year at a time. Each time the responsible medical officer (RMO) wishes to renew a detention beyond those periods, he or she must justify it to the district health authority, having first consulted another professional involved in the treatment. Otherwise the RMO and the district health authority can discharge the patient at any time. The patient has a right to apply to a Mental Health Review Tribunal (MHRT) once during each of those periods. The Tribunal is composed of an independent lawyer, psychiatrist and someone with special skills in social services. The patient's nearest relative (see the box on p. 80) is entitled to discharge patients detained under this section but must give 72 hours' notice. During that time the RMO can overrule the relative. However, if the doctor does overrule it, the nearest relative has a right to apply to the Tribunal.

The 'hospital order' allows a court to send a defendant to hospital rather than punish him or her. If this happens, the patient is treated as if detained under a treatment order except that there is no right of appeal in the first six months. This means that the doctor could discharge someone soon after admission even though a serious criminal offence had been committed. However, the Crown courts can also impose a 'restriction order', which means that only the Home Secretary, who receives advice from his or her own officers, and the Tribunal can discharge the patient. (When hearing applications in these cases the Tribunal has to consider different rules.) Patients can also be transferred from prisons under a 'transfer order' and a 'restriction direction' can be added to these orders to restrict the RMO's powers to discharge.

These orders can only be used with patients who have a mental illness, psychopathic disorder, mental impairment or severe mental impairment. So most patients with mental handicaps cannot be detained for prolonged periods. Where the patient is said to have a mental impairment or psychopathic disorder, a treatability test must be considered. It must be shown that the patient's condition will be alleviated by, or at least will not deteriorate under, the treatment to be provided. 'Treatment' includes nursing care and everything that is provided under medical supervision. The patient's disorder must also make it appropriate to detain him or her for treatment in hospital. Detention is not justified if the patient could be treated, just as well, in the community. The treatment must be necessary for the patient's health or to protect others.

Can patients be detained for short assessment periods?

Sometimes the patient's exact diagnosis and needs will not be known. To be admitted under an 'assessment order' the patient may have any mental disorder, but it must be of a nature or degree that warrants detention for assessment. It must be necessary for the patient's health or to protect others. Once made, this order authorises the detention of the patient for up to 28 days. That should be sufficient time for clinicians to decide whether longer-term detention is necessary and to make a more specific diagnosis of the disorder. The patient can apply to a Mental Health Review Tribunal within the first 14 days of detention. A similar problem can arise when people appear before the courts. Their diagnosis and treatment needs, if any, may be uncertain. So the courts have similar powers. Courts can remand a defendant to a hospital for a medical report (section 35) or for treatment (section 36). These orders also only last for 28 days but can be extended, for a similar period, up to a maximum of 12 weeks.

Who can make these orders?

Hospital and remand orders are made by the criminal courts after receiving two supporting medical reports. Only a Crown court can make a restriction order. The assessment and treatment orders also require two supporting medical reports. One should be given by a doctor acknowledged by the district health authority as especially skilled in the diagnosis of mental disorder and one should have prior knowledge of the patient. This points to, but does not require, a psychiatrist and the patient's general practitioner. They must examine the patient.

The application for a treatment or assessment order must be made by the nearest relative or an 'approved' social worker. The social worker should consult the nearest relative about assessment orders and must, if reasonably practicable, consult them before making a treatment order. The nearest relative can prevent a hospital order but not an assessment order being made. If the objection to a hospital order is considered unreasonable, the social worker must ask a county court to relieve the nearest relative of his or her rights. An application made by a social worker who is not actually approved, or a relative who is not the nearest, will be an invalid detention. Once the application, based upon the medical reports, has been made, the applicant can authorise anyone, such as an ambulance officer or nurse, to take or assist in taking a patient to a hospital and detaining him or her there.

Can patients be detained in emergencies?

It can be difficult to get two doctors to a patient quickly and it may be unwise to wait. So a patient may be detained, in an 'emergency' for up to 72 hours where the nearest relative's or approved social worker's application is only based on one medical report. Within those 72 hours the patient can be seen by a specialist and a fuller social report prepared. The emergency order may then be discharged or the patient detained under another power.

If a police officer thinks that a person is mentally disordered in a place to which the public have access and is in need of immediate care or control, he or she may remove that person to a place of safety for up to 72 hours if it is necessary and in the individual's interests. The definition of place of safety includes hospitals and police stations. During that period, the individual is to be seen by an approved social worker and doctor, who may decide to use another section to move the individual to hospital for a further period. The individual need not have committed any offence.

Can voluntary inpatients be detained?

Most inpatients in mental illness and mental handicap units are voluntary patients. They may not be there voluntarily in the sense, for example, that they have been told that they may and will be detained unless they stay, but they are, in law, entitled to discharge themselves and leave. If those patients try to leave they can sometimes be detained. There are other patients who come from their homes to wards and other areas for treatment during the day, who cannot be detained if they try to leave. There are also patients in general wards who may have mental disorders. Sometimes these patients can be detained.

If a voluntary inpatient's doctor thinks that an application ought to be made for the patient to be compulsorily admitted, but only for treatment for a mental disorder, he or she may provide a written report to the health authority under section 5(2). This order lasts for up to 72 hours during which time other orders might be made. The patient's doctor may nominate one other doctor on the hospital's staff to have these powers in his or her absence. This can be the duty doctor. The patient must be admitted to the same hospital but mental disorder wards are not specified. So a patient on a general ward could be detained as could a patient, after having been admitted via casualty, after taking, for example, an overdose.

What if the doctor cannot get to the ward fast enough to make an order?

An inpatient may decide to leave when there are no doctors available to sign the forms. They may act in an aggressive manner or threaten to commit crimes. Nurses can act immediately. Any person, including nurses, may use such force as is reasonably necessary to prevent a crime, including protecting themselves and others. This is specified in section 3 of the Criminal Law Act 1967. The power is to prevent, and not to punish, a crime. This covers attempted crimes where the patient has done something more than merely preparatory towards committing a crime. So talking about or threatening a crime like theft will rarely be sufficient because that is not more than preparatory. However, putting someone, including nurses and other patients, in fear of immediate physical danger is a crime in itself (assault) and thus would justify some preventative action.

Nevertheless, leaving or threatening to leave a hospital, or to commit suicide, are not crimes. So the 1967 Act cannot be used with them. Section 5(4) of the 1983 Act provides an alternative remedy. If a 'prescribed nurse' thinks that a patient is suffering from any form of mental disorder to such a degree that it is necessary for the patient's health or safety or for others' protection that the patient is immediately restrained from leaving hospital, and yet it is not practicable to get a doctor present to make a section 5(2) order, she or he may record the facts in writing and detain the patient. 'Prescribed nurse' means those nurses registered in parts 3 and 5 of the professional register as being trained in the nursing of people with mental illness or mental handicap respectively. The patient must be receiving treatment for mental disorder as an inpatient, so this procedure should not be used with patients arriving in casualty or arriving in a mental disorder ward but who have not been formally admitted or are not yet receiving treatment. The procedure allows the patient to be detained for up to six hours or until the RMO, or nominated deputy, arrives on the ward when he or she may make a report detaining the patient for 72 hours, during which time an assessment or treatment order may be made.

It should be noted that the 1983 Act's special rules on the compulsory treatment of patients, discussed below, do not apply to patients who have only been detained by a nurse. Similarly, they do not apply to patients detained just for 72 hours where there has only been one medical recommendation. So, if compulsory treatment of a patient is considered in these circumstances, for example sedation, then it must be justified under the general law.

Do nurses have a special role in the detention of patients under the Mental Health Act?

Applications for detention are normally made by nearest relatives or approved social workers and based upon medical recommendations. While nurses may advise doctors and provide them with reports, they have no official role in the detention process, except under the special six-hour power. They may be the person consulted before a long-term treatment order is renewed but consulting does not require the nurse's support. They may have important practical roles in ensuring that the paperwork is correct. They may, for example, be designated by the health authority as the person to receive doctor's reports, under the emergency procedures, after normal hours. They will receive applications from nearest relatives who wish to discharge patients detained under a treatment order and will have to make quick decisions about whether and how to act if a voluntary patient decides to leave. They are also likely to be delegated responsibility for section 132 of the Act, which requires the health authority to take such steps as are practicable to ensure that detained patients understand the grounds for their detention and their rights to apply to a Tribunal. That information must be given orally and in writing as soon as practicable after detention.

How can nurses recognise the patient's nearest relative?

Some mistakes, for example an inaccurate diagnosis, can be rectified later and do not invalidate a detention. However, other mistakes cannot be altered and they could create a case of false imprisonment. Problems are particularly possible with applications made by nearest relatives. The legal definition of this person is very unusual although precise. In many cases the co-residents of the patient in long-stay residential accommodation will be the nearest relative even over genuine relatives! The table should help find this elusive legal person. Hopefully, nurses will not often be embroiled in these unnecessarily complicated rules, although they could be when dealing with patients' relatives. It will have been noticed that it is a very different idea from next of kin.

Finding a detained patient's nearest relative

First discover all the people who count as 'relatives'

These are: (a) husband or wife, (b) son or daughter, (c) father or mother, (d) brother or sister, (e) grandparent, (f) grandchild, (g) uncle or aunt, (h) nephew or niece. Relationships of half-blood are treated the same as whole blood. Illegitimate children are treated as only their mother's child. 'Husband and wife' includes unmarried couples unless there is also a legal partner who still counts as a relative. And any person with whom the patient has been ordinarily residing for at least five years (or had when detained) is to be treated as a relative at the end of the list. This will include many homosexual relationships but 'residing with' is so broad that it will include people living together in communities or institutions such as hospitals and Part III accommodation.

Discount certain relatives

Exclude those not ordinarily resident in the UK, Channel Islands or Isle of Man. Exclude spouses permanently separated by agreement or court order and those who have or have been and remain deserted. Exclude those under 18 years at the relevant time except when the spouse or parent of the patient. Exclude those who have a conviction for incest with a person under 18 years.

Find the 'nearest' relative

Regrettably, section 26 gives two tests that can lead to different results. One rule states that the relative highest in the list, that is closest to (a), is the nearest relative. The other rule states that any relative with whom the patient was ordinarily resident at the time of detention is the nearest relative. This means that those people who have resided with the patient for five years will often

►

be the nearest relative although they cannot be where a married spouse who has not been separated or deserted still exists. It is thought that this second rule should be used first and then the other rule used if there still remain several relatives. And if there are still several equally close relatives left then the eldest is the nearest for the law's purposes.

Check whether the nearest relative has assigned the rights

Nearest relatives are entitled, under the regulations, to assign their rights to another person. The person who appears to be the nearest relative should be asked whether the rights have been assigned.

Can patients, with a mental disorder, be treated against their will?

Generally, as was explained in Chapter 5, adult patients may not be treated against their will. However, patients may reject treatment because of their disorder or have difficulties in assessing the issues when deciding whether to consent. So the 1983 Act authorises some compulsory treatment for detained patients. It distinguishes four levels of seriousness of treatment with accompanying degrees of protection for the patient. Where psychosurgery or the surgical implantation of hormones to reduce male sex drive is proposed, the patient must consent and an independent doctor approve. This rule also applies to voluntary patients. Where electro-convulsive therapy or medication, by any means, is proposed then either the patient must consent or an independent doctor approve. This rule does not apply where medication is proposed and the patient has not yet been detained for three months. During this 'trial period' neither consent nor a second opinion is necessary. When independent doctors are brought into the hospital for these purposes, they must consult two people professionally involved in the treatment of the patient, one of whom must be a nurse. As it is only a consultation, the nurse's advice can be ignored. If treatment is urgently required, then these rules can be set aside. (Section 62 specifies what 'urgent' means and the kinds of treatment that can be imposed in different circumstances of urgency.) Otherwise any treatment may be imposed upon a detained patient. This includes, for example, behaviour modification.

These special statutory powers only authorise treatment for a mental disorder. Thus they could justify use of a stomach pump on a patient who took a drug overdose while disordered but not where the patient is merely dependent upon drugs since that is expressly outside the definition of 'mental disorder'. They do not authorise abortions or sterilisation operations on women with learning difficulties. And the statutory powers only apply where the patient is detained under an order with two medical recommendations. The House of Lords decided in 1989 that medical care, including sterilisations and abortions, may be carried out on a person with a mental handicap who is unable to give a valid consent if the clinicians believe it is in the patient's best interests. They relied upon the common law. Court approval is not essential.

Can patients be compulsorily treated in the community?

Under section 7 of the 1983 Act, a patient with a mental illness, psychopathic disorder, mental impairment or severe mental impairment, may be admitted to guardianship rather than hospital. This, too, is based upon two medical recommendations and lasts, initially, for six months like section 3 hospital treatment orders. The guardian must be acceptable to the local social services authority. The guardian has three powers: (a) to require the patient to reside at a particular place, (b) to require him or her to attend specified places for medical treatment, occupation, education or training, and (c) to require that access is allowed to a doctor, approved social worker or other specified person. These powers are rather limited. While patients under guardianship may be returned to the place where they are to reside, there is no authority to force them to stay there. The power is to require a patient to attend for treatment, and so on, and that does not authorise any use of force. Not allowing access to a patient is an offence (under section 129) but force may not be used to gain access. However, in practice, many people may believe that the guardian has these practical powers and acquiesce. Patients under a guardianship order cannot be treated against their will; the sections of the 1983 Act authorising compulsory treatment can only be used with inpatients. While patients can be given leave from hospital during their period of detention, they cannot be given trial leave and treated compulsorily in the community.

Can patients sue nurses?

Section 139 of the 1983 Act imposes restrictions upon patients suing nurses and others (but not health authorities or the Department of Health) involved in their treatment. Patients must get permission from a High Court judge before they can bring their case. The Court will give permission if there are issues that deserve fuller inquiry and debate. If permission is granted, the patient must show, in addition to his or her case, that the acts were performed 'in bad faith or without reasonable care'. Staff cannot be prosecuted in the criminal courts without the permission of the Director of Public Prosecutions. These are significant protections, although applications for judicial review can be made without permission being first granted. However, it remains unclear whether this section covers detained patients only.

Because patients are in a relatively powerless position, a Mental Health Act Commission has been established with special powers and duties to protect their interests. The MHAC provides the doctors who can give the necessary second opinions for certain forms of treatment. They also visit hospitals and can hear complaints and comments from patients. They publish reports commending good practices.

Can nurses protect a mentally disordered person who is being cheated?

The right to manage our own finances is jealously guarded. However, because of their disorder or learning difficulty, some people may make unwise decisions about their property. This could leave them open to exploitation. If they voluntarily deprive themselves of resources then, under rules concerning means tests for income maintenance and social services, they can be treated as if they still have them. Consequently, their inability to manage their property may prevent them moving from hospital to more appropriate accommodation. The range of alternative ways of managing the long-term financial affairs of people with mental disorders is discussed in Chapter 8 in relation to elderly people. Here the discussion will be limited to the action nurses can take in an emergency.

Contracts are agreements between two or more people to do or exchange something lawful. The law emphasises the form of the agreement rather than its content. The courts will enforce contracts even if one of the parties is mentally disordered. It does not matter that the contract is unfair between the parties. However, there is an exception where one party knows that the other is disordered. That he or she ought to know is not enough; actual knowledge is required and this is difficult to prove. Even where one person appears to have a disorder or disability the other must know that it affects his or her ability to contract.

Nurses knowing that a patient is making such a contract could inform the other person of the patient's disorder so that the other person knows and the contract can later be invalidated. However, in some circumstances, this could breach duties of confidence. Alternatively, a nurse could apply to the Court of Protection for an emergency order. (The Court and its procedures are discussed in Chapter 8.) This would require compelling evidence of both the disorder and the emergency, but once granted, the Court is empowered to deal with the patient's property. Finally, if someone is making false statements, deliberately or recklessly ('reckless' is discussed shortly), to obtain property from a patient or to get the patient to do something for them, then that person may be committing or attempting the offence of dishonestly obtaining property or services by deception under the Theft Acts of 1967 and 1978. In such cases, the police should be informed.

While the courts will not interfere just because the contract is unfair they will interfere where the relationship between the contracting parties is unfair. If one party has 'undue' influence over another person, who has not received independent advice, the courts may set the contract aside under the rule of 'undue influence'. Nurses are likely to be regarded as having undue influence over their patients. So any nurse who buys, for example, a car for a bargain price from a patient (whether or not mentally disordered) may find the contract set aside. His or her employer should also have rules covering such cases. Patients should be advised to go to solicitors in such cases. If the contract is with nurses or others in the private residential or nursing care services, the owners and managers of those services should be reported to the local social services department or district health authority responsible for registering them. There are directives discouraging contracts between staff and patients in the private and voluntary sector. The health or local authority could take steps to de-register the home.

Can mentally disordered people be prosecuted for crimes?

Mentally disordered people are not exempt from the criminal law. However, there will often be concern whether a court appearance and punishment will benefit anyone, so prosecutions are comparatively rare. This may be an unwise policy, as individuals may be associated with criminal behaviour without ever having a chance to clear their name or to blame others. The definition, in the 1983 Act, of 'mental impairment' and 'psychopathic disorder', which can lead to long-term detention, specifies that the patient must be associated with or have caused abnormally aggressive or seriously irresponsible behaviour. This would frequently amount to a crime. Not prosecuting can imply a belief that patients are like children and not fully responsible for their acts, which is contrary to most nursing and modern service philosophies.

Virtually all crimes have two essential ingredients, (a) the prohibited behaviour (called the 'actus reus'), such as 'causing damage to another's property', and (b) a state of mind or quality of behaviour (called the 'mens rea') such as 'intention' or 'recklessness'. The defendant must have caused the prohibited behaviour with that state of mind or quality of behaviour. If a person did not intend to do the prohibited act, because of a mental disorder or for any other reason, then he or she cannot be guilty of any crime, such as murder or theft, which requires intention. However, if a person performs an act that other reasonable people would regard as obviously risky, which the defendant did not regard as risky because of mental disorder, then he or she will be guilty of any crime such as criminal damage that can be committed, with only recklessness. 'Intention' requires the individual to will, want, plan, etc. but 'recklessness' has been defined as either deliberately taking a risk or doing something that ordinary people would realise was obviously risky. So a patient who did not intend to take another's property, because of his or her disorder, will not be guilty of theft, which can only be committed intentionally. However, a patient who did not intend to cause criminal damage and did not realise there was a risk of harm, could be guilty of criminal damage as that can be committed intentionally or recklessly. And, in law, it is possible to be reckless if the patient did not realise but reasonable people without disorders would have realised there was a risk.

Do people with mental disorders have a defence to criminal liability?

If the defendant caused the 'actus reus', and had the state of mind required, he or she may still use any legal defence that is available. There are two particular defences relating to mental disorder. The McNaghten Rules govern the defence of 'insanity'. They require that the defendant had (1) a defect of reason (2) due to a disease of the mind that either (3a) led to him or her not knowing the nature and quality of the act or (3b) if he or she did understand them then he or she did not know that the acts were wrong. The tests are clinically outmoded although they were radical when first formulated. For example, the House of Lords recently decided that psychomotor epilepsy was included. However, cases where an individual knows what he or she is doing and that it is wrong, but cannot control his or her urges, are excluded. Defendants who successfully plead insanity are found not guilty but are then detained at Her Majesty's pleasure, often for longer than the maximum prison sentence available for the offence. So the defence of insanity is rarely used even though available for all offences.

The defence of diminished responsibility is only available to people charged with murder. If successful, the defendant will be found not guilty of murder but guilty of manslaughter. Judges must impose life imprisonment for murder but have complete discretion with manslaughter. The defence requires that the individual suffered from 'such abnormality of mind . . . as substantially impaired his mental responsibility for his acts'. There is also a defence of automatism, which requires that the person has no control over his or her body. It is a complete defence to all crimes. This might appear appropriate for some people with mental disorders but if the evidence points towards a 'defect of reason' and 'disease of the mind', as was said to be the case with psychomotor epilepsy, the judges will require that the defendant also pleads insane. At this stage, defendants tend to prefer to drop the defence.

Patients may use any other defence that is appropriate. Some, such as being drunk or under the influence of drugs, are only defences to crimes where the 'mens rea' is, exclusively, stated in terms of intention. The idea is that the person who is sufficiently drunk or under the influence of drugs will be incapable of intending the prohibited behaviour. So these defences are not so much special rules as examples of the general rule that if a defendant does not have the essential 'mens rea' then he or she will not have committed a crime. If, as a result of the mental disorder, a patient did not intend the prohibited act there will have been no crime. However, if the crime can be committed with a 'mens rea' less than intention, a crime may have been committed.

Can patients be prosecuted even when disordered?

Some defendants can be at a considerable disadvantage when charged with crimes. They may, for example, lack alibis or resources to seek evidence that helps them. They may simply forget what happened at the relevant time or they might have then been or now be mentally disordered.

There are special procedures if the charge is one that can be tried, as most can be, by a magistrates' court. Section 37 of the Mental Health Act 1983 provides that if a defendant could not be guilty, because his or her mental disorder prevented him or her having the 'mens rea' for the offence, the magistrates can still make a hospital order. If they could not do this, the defendant would have to be found 'not guilty' and no hospital order could be considered.

Unfortunately, it means that any defence the patient may have may go unheard. That the patient took some articles does not mean, for example, that he or she intended to take them, which is essential before there is theft. This procedure can be used even when the patient is so disordered that he or she cannot enter a meaningful plea of 'guilty' or 'not guilty'.

The above procedure is not available before the Crown courts, where the more serious offences are tried. If there is concern that a defendant is too mentally disordered to properly be involved in the proceedings, the test being whether he or she can properly instruct his or her lawyer in making a defence, a special jury is established to decide this preliminary question of capacity.

Are nurses entitled to restrict mentally disordered patients' sexuality?

People with mental disorders are entitled to the same rights and protections as others until a specific law provides otherwise. So the law concerning rape, homosexual acts, indecent exposure, and so on, applies to them as much as others. The right to express ourselves sexually, in socially acceptable ways, is highly regarded. Yet within health and social services, people with mental disorders are frequently discouraged, directly and indirectly, from expressing their sexuality. Nurses and others often find it a very difficult subject because so many different values and personal experiences are involved. However, patients' civil rights and opportunities for pleasure and growth are also involved.

Important concepts in this area of law are 'unlawful sexual inter-course' and 'consent'. Here 'unlawful' does not mean criminal but 'outside the bounds of marriage'. Many acts that could be criminal outside of marriage, like rape, are lawful within marriage. (Although not considered as rape, violent non-consensual intercourse within marriage will still constitute a criminal offence.) And 'consent', where sexual offences are concerned, can be interpreted differently to other areas. A person only consenting under a threat of force or under pressure and without an easy option, may be regarded as not consenting. For example, a person who is told: 'Unless you sleep with me I'll see that your discharge is delayed', is likely to be treated as not consenting if they should comply.

There are several offences of having unlawful sexual intercourse with a woman who is a 'defective', or arranging it. Similarly, it is an offence for a man to commit an act of gross indecency on another man, whatever age, who is 'severely subnormal'. These are crimes irrespective of whether the individual consents. The law is deeming them incapable of consent. Here 'defective' and 'severely sub-normal' refer to part of the definition of 'severe mental impairment' in section 1 of the Mental Health Act 1983. The individual must have severely impaired intelligence and social functioning. There is no requirement of association with inappropriate behaviour. While intelligence quotients may be relatively stable and not amenable to change by nurses, the same cannot be said of levels of social functioning. If such a patient wishes to express his or her sexuality, nurses could devise ways of increasing his or her social functioning so that he or she no longer falls within the definition of 'defective'. Indeed, in the light of professional and other duties to enhance the individual's life experiences and to avoid problems such as frustration and socially inappropriate sexual conduct (such as exhibitionism), nurses ought to implement programmes to increase 'social functioning' levels and socially appropriate and individually rewarding sex-education programmes.

It is often a defence to these crimes that the other person did not know, and had no reason to suspect, that the other was 'defective' or 'severely subnormal'. If nurses are concerned that someone is likely to exploit a severely mentally impaired person, they could give that person reason to suspect the other's disorder. This would, as the nurse could explain, prevent them having this defence.

It is an offence for male staff, including managers, to have 'un-lawful' sexual intercourse with women being treated for mental disorder or with any woman subject to their guardianship under the 1983 Act. These offences are not limited to women deemed to be 'defectives'. And, in addition to the criminal laws, there will be professional rules and employers' rules about what is unacceptable conduct. In practice, much attention will be paid to relationships that are exploitative.

How can nurses respond to patients' sexuality without fear of legal liability?

These rules can give nurses very difficult problems. On the one hand they appreciate that sexuality is an important part of the whole person and an important potentially pleasurable experience. However, it is also subject to many taboos and conflicting attitudes in the general population. Patients' sexuality should not simply be ignored. Not being able or allowed to express themselves may cause considerable distress. It may lead to them acting in socially unacceptable ways that delay integration into a caring community. They may commit crimes. If harm is reasonably foreseeable from nurses failing to provide appropriate services, they may be liable in the law of negligence for failing to take proper precautions. The box below suggests steps that can help prevent liability.

Responsibility when responding to patients' sexuality

Encourage marriage

If a couple are married their intercourse cannot be unlawful, although it may still be a crime, if for example it involves violence. To be a valid marriage, both parties must have a basic understanding of its nature.

Promote skills training

A patient may be legally 'defective'. Acting so that he or she can no longer be regarded as having severely impaired social functioning will mean that he or she no longer fits within the definition of 'defective' and is therefore able, if an adult, to consent.

Note that failure to provide services may cause harm

It may be reasonably foreseeable that a failure to provide services will cause harm. So there is a duty to respond and try to prevent those harms. Employers should be reminded of their responsibilities to both patients and staff and be encouraged to provide training and develop policies that could incorporate risk-taking strategies.

Emphasise patient-centred objectives

To discourage any suggestion of paternalism or exploitation, the services provided should meet the needs that the patient perceives.

Emphasise consent

Even where there are communication problems it should be possible to show that a patient has understood what is happening and freely approves.

CHAPTER 8

People who are elderly

A large and increasing proportion of patients in our hospitals are elderly. Usually their age will be of no legal relevance to their treatment or life-style. Nevertheless, several legal problems are associated, although not exclusively, with old age. These include:

1 Unhygienic homes. Very occasionally some people live in conditions that harm their own or threaten others' health. There are powers to remove such people from their homes.

2 Managing property and money. Some people are unable, because of mental disorder, to manage their financial affairs. These problems are often associated with old age. While few people, however wise, may wish to prepare for being mentally disordered and incapable there are practical and individualised ways of preventing many problems from arising.

3 Special housing needs. With increasing problems of mobility some elderly people have special housing needs. Some people in hospitals might be better placed in such housing. The private sector provides some special housing where special laws apply.

These areas of law are not limited to elderly people. Being elderly may mean pensions are payable and there is, sometimes, entitlement to special housing. However, it does not lead to any special legal status in the sense that mental disorder can. The general law of negligence, for example, still applies. Elderly people are still entitled to refuse or consent to treatment. There may be differences in practice, such as a reluctance to take risks or reduced priority for treatment. The legality of any such differences would have to be decided by applying general principles.

The law governing residential and nursing homes is not limited to units designed for elderly people. Indeed the Act that regulates nursing homes also applies to private acute hospitals. The special laws on managing patients' property and finance depend upon proof of mental disorder and have nothing, directly, to do with elderly people. However, in practice, these legal issues are particularly relevant to elderly people. Most people subject to the

Court of Protection, which supervises the property of people who are incapable because of a mental disorder, are elderly.

Can elderly people who are living in unsafe or unhygienic circumstances be moved from them?

The ways in which some people, diagnosed as having a mental disorder, can be detained in hospitals or, through guardianship orders, can be told where to reside are described in Chapter 7. The same procedures can be used with people who are elderly and have a mental disorder. Section 47 of the National Assistance Act 1948 provides another procedure. The object is to secure 'the necessary care and attention of people who (a) are suffering from grave chronic disease or, being aged, infirm or physically incapacitated, are living in insanitary conditions, and (b) are unable to devote to themselves, and are not receiving from other persons, proper care and attention'. Clearly, it is not limited to elderly people. Where the patient has a 'grave chronic disease', unlike the other categories, there is no need to prove insanitary conditions.

A community physician must certify, in writing to the local authority, that it is necessary in the individual's interests or to prevent ill-health or serious nuisance to others, to move the person from his or her home. The authority applies to a magistrates' court, which may authorise removal to a suitable hospital or other place at a convenient distance. The order authorises detention for three months, which the court can keep renewing for similar periods. The patient can only apply for the order to be revoked after six weeks. Any expenses incurred through not placing the patient in a hospital or (social services') Part III accommodation may be recovered from the patient.

The patient, and the managers of the unit where the person will be placed, must be given seven days' notice of an application. In urgent cases, this could prove a stumbling block. However, the National Assistance (Amendment) Act 1951 provides that, if the community physician and another doctor certify it is urgent, an application can be made to just one magistrate if necessary, without giving notice or the patient being represented. Such an order only lasts three weeks but, during this time, a three-month order can be sought.

The patients involved with these laws are likely to be friendless, otherwise they would rarely fit the legal definition. The powers may be administratively useful but constitute a major loss of civil rights. Little publicity or debate attaches to them as such patients are unlikely to appeal to higher courts and friends are unlikely to intervene on their behalf as they might be asked why they are not providing the help.

Can elderly people give their property and income to someone else to manage for them?

Any person may choose to have another person administer and look after their property. The rights of the people involved will depend upon the agreement they make. If both parties benefit, for example one is paid a fee and the other receives a service, then there will usually be a contract. Contracts can be very useful devices for specifying rights and relationships. Even if problems were never contemplated, so that there was little discussion about the details, the courts can imply terms and protect people. In the absence of a contract, there are few rights; the neighbour's promise to visit, the relative's financial support and the public's charity cannot be enforced. Having contractual rights also gives increased status – it is felt to be one of the benefits of private health over the NHS. Any patient making arrangements for their property, or affecting their future, should be encouraged to make a contract.

People may give their property away. Here there is no contract to enforce as there is no exchange of benefits. Once given, there is no right to get it back. (If the giver happens to be mentally disordered then, as discussed in Chapter 7, an emergency order may be sought from the Court of Protection.) However, they can 'attach strings'. When one person passes property, which includes money, to another but, explicitly or implicitly, imposes restrictions on how or for whom it is to be used, a trust is created. The ownership of the property passes to the other, called a trustee, but the courts will require the trustee to meet the restrictions imposed. So people who do not wish to, or fear they will be unable to, manage their property when elderly, could create a trust to prevent problems. Solicitors should be employed to avoid difficulties. Creating trusts in an informal or secret way is very risky as problems often result over what was intended. In addition, they are rarely successful when the objective is to avoid a means test for social services' charges or social security.

Can elderly people appoint someone to administer their property if they should become incapable?

A problem occurs when elderly people have property but become mentally disordered and incapable of managing it. Sometimes patients are physically fit to move to a nursing home and have the money to pay for it but there are problems in getting access to that money because the individual is incapable of managing it. In the last resort, the Court of Protection can appoint a receiver with the power to manage the patient's property. However, this can be expensive, impersonal and discourage rehabilitation. The Enduring Powers of Attorney Act 1985 provides a much better answer but it depends upon people acting before they become disordered.

We can ordinarily appoint other people to make legal decisions, say sell a house or manage our bank account, on our behalf. To do this we give them a power of attorney. Until we cancel it that person can make decisions that are legally binding on us and others. The attorney must abide by any restrictions specified. They can be paid or unpaid, official people like bank managers and solicitors or friends and relatives. The donor, the person who makes the power, remains the owner of the property, and in charge in that he or she can cancel the power and can control it by imposing restrictions on it. For example, an attorney may be authorised to mortgage but not to sell a house. So if nurses know that an attorney has been appointed, they could investigate to see whether he or she is authorised to meet, for example, nursing home fees for a patient.

However, there is a catch! People who are mentally disordered and incapable cannot make new ordinary powers of attorney. Furthermore, existing powers come to an end as soon as the donor becomes disordered and incapable. To avoid these problems an enduring power of attorney must be created under the 1985 Act. To ensure that everyone realises the significance of making an enduring power they must be made in a formal way on special documents, witnessed and signed. The document explains that this power will continue in force if the donor should become mentally incapable.

Once made, an enduring power can operate as an ordinary power or be held in abeyance. However, just as soon as the donor starts to become mentally disordered the attorney must apply to the Court of Protection to have the enduring power registered. The Court will have notices sent to certain relatives, other attorneys and, usually, the donor. These people may make comments, which the Court will consider. If there are no comments or the Court nevertheless, after investigation, decides not to invalidate the power or for other reasons not to enforce it, the Court must register the power. While formal notices only go to specified relatives, anyone can send in comments at any stage and the Court can review the power and cancel it at any stage. During the weeks when notices are being sent out, the attorney has some powers, which can, if necessary, be increased by the Court. The attorney can, for example, ensure that the donor, who may now be a patient, has income to pay for accommodation.

What steps could nurses take to ensure that enduring powers of attorney are not abused?

The biggest 'abuse' may be not knowing how enduring powers of attorney can help! If no power is made, or it is only an ordinary power, then the Court of Protection's receivership powers may have to be used. They are impersonal, bureaucratic and expensive. All nurses should encourage patients, and prospective patients, to make wills and enduring powers. That will increase patients' control of their futures and reduce future problems. It should not be left to nurses working in the psychogeriatric services as their patients may already be legally incompetent. Nurses should advise patients to contact their own solicitors, who have ready access to the forms and who can incorporate the individual's wishes into the document. Nurses should not draft legal documents on behalf of patients and should not become attorneys for their patients. Employers would not approve and it is most unwise to get into a position where motives can be doubted, such as wanting access to a patient's money for personal profit.

Another 'abuse' could be failure to use the potential of enduring powers. Patients should be encouraged to write protections into their power. Unless they specify otherwise, a general enduring power may be created. This will give the attorney very wide powers including the right to use the patient's property to support relatives and others. Nevertheless, the patient can specify which relatives and charities are to be supported and which not, which property can be sold and which mortgaged, that the funds may be used to buy a house but not to pay nursing home fees, or whatever. These restrictions may be avoided in exceptional cases as the Court of Protection can cancel a power and use its receivership powers instead. However, it is the right to stipulate individual wishes in the power that enables this procedure to be so much more personal and individual than other procedures.

The Court of Protection does not police enduring powers to ensure that attorneys do not abuse their positions and are not incompetent. They rely on people like nurses reporting suspected abuses to the Court, who can then inquire and act. Nurses could also advise patients to suggest that their solicitor inserts a term that requires that a copy of the power is filed with, say, the Director of Social Services. Unless it is possible to check the terms of the power, it will be difficult to know whether there are abuses. At no stage in the proceedings are psychiatrists, nurses or others formally consulted as to whether the donor actually is mentally disordered. So a term could be written into the power requiring the attorney to arrange that regular medical reports are submitted to the Court. If a patient recovers sufficiently to be legally capable of managing his or her property, he or she can formally cancel the enduring power. This might be unwise if a relapse is possible and a new enduring power is not made in the interval. Alternatively, the attorney may be persuaded to allow the patient control of his or her property during that time without altering the formal legal position.

Attorneys can retire at any stage by giving notice to the court. Substitutes cannot be appointed by anyone. So the effect of an attorney being pressurised too much could be his or her retirement, with the consequence that the power ends and the Court of Protection has to use its receivership powers. Patients should be careful about whom they appoint. They should be likely to survive the patient and should be competent to manage the kind of work involved. It is possible to appoint a solicitor, bank official or similar person together with a relative. In this way technical skills and individual attention can be married. However, the specially skilled person, at least, will expect and is entitled to be paid.

What is 'mental incapacity' in the law and why is it significant?

For an enduring power of attorney to be valid the donor must have been legally competent to make it. If he or she was not competent at the time it was made then it will be invalid. So what is meant by 'legal incapacity' could be crucial. There are different tests for 'mental incapacity' depending upon whether enduring powers or receivership orders are involved. It is possible, in law, for a person to be incapable of managing his or her property and affairs so that the Court of Protection could make a receivership order and yet still be able to make a valid enduring power of attorney. To make a valid enduring power, the donor must understand the nature and effect of what he or she is doing. The High Court has given four practical tests for guidance. Does the donor understand:

1 that the attorney will get complete authority over the donor's property and affairs;
2 that the attorney will be able to do anything with the property that the donor could have done;
3 that the attorney's powers continue during the donor's in-capacity; and
4 that, after becoming incapable, the donor will not be able to revoke the power without the Court's permission?

If the donor is going to restrict the attorney's powers then he or she, in order to be legally capable of making that particular enduring power, must understand the nature and effect of those restrictions. The four practical tests would be applied to those restrictions. So a person with a degree of mental disorder and difficulty in understanding and managing his or her property, may still be able to make a valid power. Nevertheless, the more detailed the restrictions the individual wants, the less likely it will be for that person to be able to understand the nature and effect of them so as to make it a valid enduring power. It would be unfortunate if the High Court's interpretation, designed to encourage use of the enduring powers laws, led to people who had delayed making their powers, being unable to write in their individualised wishes.

When does the Court of Protection use its receivership powers?

If there are no other ways of dealing with a patient's property and finances then it may be necessary to apply to the Court of Protection for a receivership order. Here the test of legal incapacity is laid down in the Mental Health Act 1983. It involves a five-part test. The patient must be: (a) incapable, (b) by reason of (c) mental disorder of (d) managing and administering his or her (e) property and affairs. The Court has agreed guidance on the meaning of this test with the British Medical Association and Royal College of Psychiatrists. A feature of the definition is its 'all or nothing' quality. Patients either come within the definition or do not, even though their degree of disorder can vary considerably. Patients may continue to be subject to the Court although they no longer satisfy the tests. This is a denial of their rights and may discourage self-respect and rehabilitation.

Nurses who are anxious to encourage their patients to exercise responsibility and make decisions for themselves, might wish to argue that some patients are still capable of managing their property. They could develop tests of capacity and use them to support their decisions to encourage patients to exercise more control and responsibility supporting them with the risk-taking analyses discussed in Chapter 3. The box below contains some suggestions.

Ways of keeping patients in charge of their property

Reorganise property and finances

Can the property and finances be reorganised so that they are easier to administer? For example, could investments in companies listed on the stock exchange be sold and the proceeds invested in a building society? The legal test is of

▶

incapacity to manage his or her property. It is easier to manage a bank account than an investment portfolio. The patient should always be advised to get independent legal or financial advice before doing anything like this. While there may be a gain in security with a bank account there could be a considerable loss of income.

Teach the patient how to manage his or her affairs

Can the patient be shown how to manage his or her property and finances? It would be improper to tell the patient which decisions to make and this would not prevent him or her from being 'incapable'. Nevertheless, training programmes, such as in concepts of value and the significance of different choices, could enable the patient to take practical charge of his or her property.

Is the patient 'incapable', or just foolish or unwise?

The law requires that the patient is 'incapable' of managing. Is the patient 'incapable' or would he or she be better described as 'foolish' or 'unwise'? Value judgments as to what people should and should not do with their property are inappropriate. The legal test requires irrational rather than inappropriate decisions. If the patient can give a rational reason for what he or she wants to do then he or she may be foolish but, in law, will be capable. However, patients should be warned that even though they deprive themselves of property they can be treated, in law, as still possessing it when they come to claim social security or social services.

Check whether the incapacity is the result of mental disorder

The incapacity must be due to mental disorder. Is it? Just being incompetent is not enough.

Check whether the patient knows what he or she possesses

Can the patient describe his or her property relatively accurately? To be capable of managing your property you should know what you possess. The standard of accuracy remains unclear as the courts have not been explicit. However, a useful test could be to ask whether most people with that kind and amount of property would know that much. For example, few of us know exactly how much we have in an account but would know whether we have a mortgage.

▶

Check whether the patient understands the legalities

Does the patient understand the basic legal rules affecting that property? For example he or she should understand that a gift involves parting with the property without a right to regain it, that contracts involve give and take. Again it is suggested that it should be the amount of information most people with that kind and amount of property would need to have to manage it without being easily exploited. They would only need to know the legal rules about the kinds of property they actually have and only in broad terms.

Is the individual being exploited?

Often the concern will be whether the individual is being exploited. Is it clear that no force or pressure is being exerted and the person is actually doing the managing for him- or herself rather than at the behest of another? If controlled by another then the individual is incapable.

Who can refer cases to the Court of Protection?

Nurses, like anyone else, can apply to the Court of Protection for a receivership order to be made affecting someone. Forms outlining that person's financial and family circumstances must be completed and a medical certificate provided by a doctor. If the Court decides that an order should be made, it will appoint someone to be receiver. This is often a relative but can be someone like the Director of Social Services or an official associated with the Court. The Court will give this person authority to do certain things with the patient's property, such as using the income to maintain the patient in private accommodation. The receiver has to justify his or her use of the money and to refer important decisions to the Court. The cost of these applications and other fees come from the patient's property.

Fraud by receivers, in the sense of deliberate misapplication of funds, is well protected against by the Court. However, receivers can also abuse their position by not using their powers actively in the patient's interest. For example, there could be a conflict of interests where a receiver is also a relative. He or she may not wish to use the patient's money to allow, say, the patient to leave hospital and enter other suitable accommodation. That would reduce the money available to be distributed on the patient's death through the will. The Master of the Court has expressed concern that most receivers are not adventurous enough in the way they exercise their powers. Nurses concerned about this could inform the Court who could respond by, for example, sending a Lord Chancellor's Visitor to investigate. In the last resort, the receiver may be removed and another appointed.

Are there other alternatives to using the Court of Protection?

Instead of receivership, the Court can make a 'short procedure order'. If the patient's property is less than £3000, or it is otherwise suitable, the Court can make one order covering virtually all that may be done with the property. This removes the need to make annual accounts and to apply to the Court to make certain decisions. The £3000 is not an absolute upper limit. If the patient's property is easy to administer, for example if it has already been collected together into manageable forms such as building society accounts, then the Court could be asked to make this sort of decision rather than the much more complicated receivership order.

If a patient's property is limited to a civil service or Ministry of Defence pension, those authorities should be approached because they have powers to pass the pension to someone to manage on the patient's behalf. If the patient receives only social security then the manager of the local office should be approached and asked to nominate an appointee. They have powers to appoint someone to receive the money and use it on behalf of the patient. These can be cheap, personalised and efficient alternatives to the other procedures. Again, abuses are possible. Nurses could protect their patients by informing the organisation concerned. These procedures rely upon the public reporting abuses.

Do any of these procedures for managing patients' property give a power to tell patients where to live or which treatment to accept?

The procedures for gaining control over a patient's property give no legal powers over the patient's body. That requires use of detention in hospital or guardianship orders, discussed in Chapter 7, or the National Assistance Acts, discussed at the beginning of this chapter. However, in practice, control over the patient's property may give considerable influence over where the patient lives. For example, being able to use the patient's property to pay for a residential care home may lead to the patient being willing to move there or, at least, not objecting. However, compulsion can only be authorised by those Acts. An elderly patient may be blocking an acute bed. He or she may have the funds to meet nursing home fees but be unable to manage them. By using any of the devices discussed above, control of the property could lead to an appropriate place being found. Nevertheless, the patient has to make the final decision.

How are elderly patients' rights protected in private-sector residential or nursing accommodation?

As was explained in Chapter 2, NHS patients have a contract neither with the NHS, nor its doctors or nurses, that they could enforce. The same is true of social services. A patient may be admitted to social services' accommodation and may be charged for those or other services after a means test. The social services' department may be obliged to provide certain services. However, there is no contract.

If an individual enters a private residential or nursing home (even if the charges are wholly met by social security payments), he or she will have two main kinds of protection, a contract and the Registered Homes Act 1984. At present, most reliance is placed upon the Act. This is unfortunate. People need to know what they are 'letting themselves in for'. Will the nursing home provide physiotherapy or chiropody services, are residents asked to leave if they become incontinent, how much notice will be given of an increase in charges? This information may be in a brochure. Nurses and others should encourage patients to ensure that this and other information is put into the contract they will have with the owners. This will often prevent problems arising and sort out some of the problems that do occur.

The Registered Homes Act is not restricted to elderly people. It provides a structure for registering and supervising the private sector residential care and nursing homes. Social services departments are responsible for supervising residential care homes. These are defined as residential accommodation with board and personal care for people who need it because of old age, disablement, past or present dependence on alcohol or drugs, or past or present mental disorder. Any place providing such accommodation for four or more non-relatives must be registered. It is a crime not to be registered. District health authorities are responsible for nursing homes, maternity homes, mental nursing homes and private hospitals. The definition refers to premises used to receive and provide nursing for people who are sick or receive medical services. It includes day services and no minimum number of patients is specified. Interesting problems can arise over the meaning of 'nursing' because if any one person in residential care receives 'nursing', that home needs to register as a nursing home or take out dual registration.

Homes wishing to be registered apply to the local social services authority and/or health authority. Negotiations take place during which the authority indicates, and finally specifies, the conditions it intends to impose upon the home's registration. Some of these are required by the statute, for example that a nursing home is under the charge of a doctor or qualified nurse, or in regulations made under the Act. Others will relate to two books of guidance about standards, *Home Life* (Centre for Policy on Ageing, 1984) for residential care homes, and *A handbook on the registration and inspection of nursing homes* (National Association of Health Authorities, 1985). The authority can add other requirements of its own, for example, it is recommended that they should specify the minimum contents of the contract the owners make with the patient or client.

Applications can be refused. Homes that have been registered can have their conditions varied or the registration can be cancelled. There is an emergency procedure where a magistrates' court can cancel registration where there is a serious risk to residents. In each case, the owners can make representations to the authority and have a right of appeal to the Registered Homes Tribunal. The Tribunal is bound by the Act and regulations but not by the books of guidance or other conditions that authorities might impose. De-registering homes causes authorities many problems as they would suddenly become responsible for meeting the needs of those patients or clients.

Residential care homes must be visited at least once a year; while nursing homes and so on must be visited at least twice a year by specially authorised officers of the authority. Visits to nursing homes will involve doctors and nurses specially authorised by their health authority. They have a right of entry. After an inspection, decisions will be made about re-registration, variation or cancellation of the registration. The minimum standards required by the Act and regulations must be met. Higher standards cannot be insisted upon by using the Act but this could be possible by encouraging residents to make, and enforce, a detailed contract.

Is it unlawful to discriminate against someone on the basis of his or her age?

This chapter should have shown that age, at the other end from childhood, is rarely relevant in our law. It is relevant to pensions but on most issues the law is blind to age. Elderly people may be more likely than others to have problems in managing their property and may make more claims on special housing, on the health and social services, but the law on those subjects is not age-specific. It involves 'mainstream' rather than special laws. Elderly people can experience discrimination, for example in receiving lower priority for treatment, but there are no laws protecting the old comparable to those relating to racial and sexual discrimination.

CHAPTER 9

People with disabilities

Patients with major disabilities and handicaps will sometimes be treated as acute patients. Obviously their legal position, as patients, will be the same as other acute services' patients during this period. Special laws only become relevant during the rehabilitation phase. These laws are designed to reduce the handicapping effect of disabilities and to ensure the coordination of services. Nurses and the health service have an important role in these patients' long-term rehabilitation. However, the principal role under the special legislation, belongs to local authorities. Therefore, the following description will aim to outline, for nurses, what the other agencies could and should be doing so that they may press those agencies. It will not be as detailed as earlier chapters as the law does not affect nurses directly.

Do disabled children have special rights during their education?

The Education Act 1981 gives local education authorities special responsibilities to discover which children have special educational needs and to respond to them. (The Act is not limited to children with physical disabilities.) A child has a learning difficulty if he or she has a significantly greater difficulty in learning than most of his or her contemporaries or his or her disability prevents or hinders use of educational facilities generally available. Some children will have their needs met by their schools being sensitive and responding appropriately. For others, there is an assessment procedure, which can lead to the education authority producing a statement of what it believes to be the child's special needs and how the authority proposes to meet them. The procedure allows parents opportunities to make comments and to challenge both the assessment of needs and any proposals for remedial action. Parents can appeal to the Secretary of State but cannot take their complaint to any special tribunal or court, except by way of judicial review as discussed in Chapter 2.

Do people with disabilities have rights to special services?

Various statutes permit health and social services authorities to provide special and additional services for people with disabilities. Nevertheless, a power is not a duty. The authorities have extensive discretion in the extent to which they respond. Section 29 of the National Assistance Act 1948, for example, allows local authorities to promote the welfare of people who are 'blind, deaf or dumb, or who suffer from mental disorder of any description and other persons who are substantially and permanently handicapped by illness, injury, or congenital deformity'. The section does not require authorities to do anything, and no individuals are given rights by the section. However, the Secretary of State may direct authorities on how they are to fulfil these duties.

Schedule 8 of the National Health Service Act allows local authorities to provide prevention, care and after-care services for people who have suffered an illness, which includes physical disability. Paragraph 3, of that Schedule, actually imposes a duty on the local authority 'to provide on such a scale as is adequate for the needs of their area' home helps where required as the result of, for example, handicaps due to illness or congenital causes. Local authorities may charge for these services and there are a range of powers for enforcing debts due to them. However, it is very difficult for individuals to enforce these duties against local authorities.

What does the Chronically Sick and Disabled Persons Act require?

The Chronically Sick and Disabled Persons Act 1970 imposes duties on various agencies, particularly local authorities. These duties are designed to ensure that the authorities consider the needs of people with disabilities but do not provide enforcement procedures or appeal procedures. Section 1 requires local authorities to know the numbers of people who may be covered by section 29 of the 1948 Act quoted above, and requires that they provide information about their services. Section 2 empowers the authority to provide various services to disabled people who come within that section 29 definition. These include practical assistance in the home, help with recreational and diversionary services, outings, help with travel, help in adapting homes for greater safety, comfort or convenience, holidays, meals and telephones. The Secretary of State might declare an authority in default if it did not provide sufficient services. The courts are reluctant to intervene, as discussed in Chapter 2, but a refusal to meet any needs, on grounds of lack of funds, might be sufficient for them to become involved. Other sections require housing authorities, planners and developers to consider the needs of people with disabilities and set up the orange badge scheme for use when parking cars.

Is it lawful to discriminate against a person with disabilities?

There are no laws that outlaw discrimination against people with disabilities in the same sense that there are laws against sexual and racial discrimination. The Disabled Persons (Employment) Act 1944 established a scheme that gave people with disabilities some preferential treatment and established a quota scheme designed to ensure that employers employed a certain proportion of people with disabilities. Its effect has been minimal and alternative schemes have been proposed. There are several schemes whereby employers can be financially supported when employing a person with disabilities or subsidised when adapting machinery and equipment. These do not give rights that the person with a disability can enforce or appeal.

Do people with disabilities have a right to a representative?

The Disabled Persons (Services Consultation and Representation) Act 1986 will establish a representation scheme for disabled people. (It was only partly in force at the time of writing.) A disabled person is someone within the definition in section 29 quoted above, which includes people with mental disorders. The person appointed will be entitled to act as a representative of the disabled person in relation to any claim for services, to accompany the disabled person to meetings about such claims, to obtain any information and see any documents that the disabled person would be entitled to see. However, the rights are limited to the occasions when the person is claiming a service that the authorities are required to provide which, as has been shown, is rarely the case.

CHAPTER 10

Children

Usually patients decide for themselves whether to accept treatment and what sort of care they want. However, children may not be sufficiently mature to make such decisions, and then it is necessary for someone else to take them. That person will usually be the child's parent. The first set of problems that have to be resolved, therefore, concern the limits of the parental right to consent to treatment for their children and issues relating to the privacy of children.

1   When does the child have the right to decide for himself?
2   Are there any sorts of treatment to which parents cannot consent?
3   Can parents veto their children's decisions?
4   How much do parents have to know about their children's treatment?

The second set of issues concern situations when the normal workings of a family have broken down. In some such cases, state intervention is necessary in order to protect children, perhaps because their parents are abusing them, but sometimes because of circumstances beyond parental control. In these cases, the usual relationship between parent and child has to be altered.

When can children decide for themselves what happens to them?

In the past, the powers of parents over their children have been very extensive; however, the modern law takes a much less authoritarian view of parenthood. Parents still have the right to make some decisions on behalf of their children while they are under 18 years of age, but it is no longer the case that before this age children automatically have no right to decide for themselves what happens to them.

By statute, a 16-year-old should be treated as an adult for the purposes of consent to treatment, so that the principles set out in Chapter 5 would apply. Although the statute does not say anything explicitly about confidentiality, the courts have assumed that, once the child is to be treated as an autonomous individual in their own right, they will have a right to information about their care being kept confidential. Even below this age, if a child has reached sufficient maturity to understand the treatment concerned, that child will be able to consent to it and should then be treated as if he or she were an adult. This was the result of the litigation in Mrs Gillick's campaign to prevent her daughters being given contraceptive advice and treatment. This is the most important relevant case and it illustrates the principles to be applied.

Mrs Gillick objected to the view of the DHSS that, in exceptional cases, doctors could advise and treat children so as to provide contraception without prior parental agreement. She argued that any consent given by a child under 16 years would be ineffective in law, and that therefore any doctor who treated a child without parental consent could be sued in trespass (see Chapter 5).

The House of Lords refused to accept this. They thought that there were some cases where children under 16 years of age could consent. It was ridiculous to suggest, they thought, that a 15-year-old child could not agree to having a grazed knee bandaged, but this would have been the result of accepting Mrs Gillick's argument. In their view, an absolute line could not be drawn. Children could validly consent to simple procedures before they could agree to complex ones. The proper test was to ask in respect of each *separate procedure* whether the child could understand what was proposed. If they could understand it, their consent to it going ahead would be valid and the parents were no longer the people to take the decision. They called this a test of maturity but pointed out that the same child could be 'mature' in respect of some procedures but 'immature' so far as others were concerned.

The main problem that this creates is that it is unclear what sort of things the child would have to be able to understand. Some of the judges suggested that it was necessary to be able to understand any moral and family issues involved and emotional implications of the treatment. Others seemed to think it was understanding about the immediate physical nature of the care that was crucial. The present writers take the view that children have only to be able to understand the physical rather than the moral aspects of the proposed care.

These last matters are probably of limited significance. The *Gillick* case concerned contraception for young girls. Most areas will be less contentious. It will usually be possible to deal with the issue as a question of the patient's ability simply to understand the basic procedures without distinguishing between different aspects. Where the child patient can understand the proposed care then they are 'mature' and have the right to be treated as if they were adults. The requirements of this are discussed in Chapter 5. If they cannot understand these explanations then, if any consent is needed, it must be sought from the parents. Where the care in question comes within the categories when no consent is needed, the parents need not be troubled for one (see Chapter 5).

What powers do parents have to decide what happens to children?

Parents can give their consent to most forms of treatment for their children, but the exact limits of this power are unclear. It has been suggested that some things, such as sterilisation, cannot be approved without going to court. The more common view is that parents are able to consent to anything that they reasonably believe to be for the child's benefit. While some medical interventions, such as removing organs for transplantation, present problems, nursing care will usually be directly for the patient's benefit and there will not normally be any difficulty in accepting parental authorisation for nursing care. This authorisation will usually be implied for routine care once the child is entrusted to the nursing staff and can be relied upon until it is withdrawn. Experimental types of care, or changes in the routine, should be checked with the parents before being used.

Where there is some doubt that parental consent would be valid it will be necessary to seek the approval of a court. An example might be where the proposed care is not only experimental, but is part of an experiment, which means that the care to be given to a child patient is not expected to benefit that patient directly at all, the purpose of the care being to discover what effects it would have, or to act as a basis for comparison. In such a case, the child patient would need to be made a 'ward of court'. This may also be necessary to prevent parents taking a decision that is not in the child's interests even though it is technically within the scope of their rights.

This was done in one case in which the parents had decided that a handicapped child should be allowed to die and had refused to consent to an operation being performed to remove an intestinal blockage. The court felt that the degree of handicap was insufficient to justify such a refusal and therefore authorised the operation. Other cases have accepted, however, that it would not be a criminal offence to allow a severely handicapped newly born child to die. Thus parents are entitled to decide to allow a severely handicapped child to die, providing that the decision to do so is taken in good faith in the interests of the child and not for some ulterior motive. Where it is felt that their decision is wrong, it can be overruled by making the child a ward of court. The parental power to take such a decision does not allow active steps to be taken solely to bring about the child's death, only omitting to provide life-sustaining treatment. As with euthanasia, acts performed in order to relieve pain, which also hasten death, will usually be permissible (see Chapter 5).

Wardship is a procedure where the child is put into the charge of the court, so that all important steps in his life must be approved in advance by the court. The court will decide what would be most to the child's benefit. This procedure was used in the controversial *Jeanette* case in the spring of 1987. The parents of a 17-year-old girl with a mental incapacity wanted her to be sterilised. As they were unsure whether the parents could authorise such an operation, the doctors made Jeanette a ward of court, and the court authorised the operation. Usually the decision would be taken by a High Court judge but because of its controversial nature, Jeanette's case was taken on appeal to the House of Lords. Any person involved with a child's care can make them a ward and, in cases where this seems necessary, nurses should seek the assistance of health authority legal departments or social services to do so.

Problems sometimes arise because parents refuse to allow care to be given. The case of the handicapped baby discussed above is an extreme example of this. Parents are entitled to use reasonable restraint in controlling children, and this means that their wishes should be recognised if they are reasonable. However, it is an offence for parents wilfully to 'neglect' their children. Failing to seek necessary medical care is 'neglect'. It is important to note, however, that parents are not required to do what is best for the child. Provided their decision is within the boundaries of what a reasonable parent would do, there is no justification in refusing to respect their wishes. This allows the recognition of minority customs so long as they are not too extreme. Even when it strays beyond this area, they will not be guilty of a criminal offence unless they were aware that they had done so. In practice, this issue usually arises in connection with positive actions rather than neglect. Courts have found parents guilty of criminal offences when they have disfigured their children with tribal markings that leave permanent scars, and Parliament has outlawed female circumcision.

The parents' rights of control and punishment will usually be delegated to those looking after a child. This makes it permissible for a nurse to use reasonable force to ensure that medication and other care is accepted by the child. What is reasonable depends on the circumstances. It is reasonable to use more force in administering necessary medicines than in making the child bath at a time convenient to the nursing staff. Nurses are entitled to rely on this implied delegation unless a parent has said that they do not want any force used. In normal circumstances, the consent of either parent is sufficient, but where one parent has indicated their disapproval of a course of action then the consent of both must be given before it is carried out.

What rights do parents have to know what is happening to their children?

This is another area where the law has never been clearly settled. The courts seem to have assumed that where a child has reached a sufficient degree of maturity to be able to consent to treatment, he will also have a right that all information concerning that treatment be kept in confidence. The scope of this right is discussed in Chapter 5. However, it is not absolute, and one of the exceptions to the obligation of confidence covers the requirements of public interest. It has been suggested that this may allow parents to be told if their children approach doctors. No court has yet considered the issue and therefore it is impossible to be certain whether such a justification would be accepted.

It is also possible that a child who is not mature enough to consent to treatment may be entitled to confidentiality. A child may be so entitled if they understand the nature of the obligation of secrecy. Therefore children should be asked whether they wish their parents to be told what is happening. If they say no, their wishes should be respected if their refusal indicates that they understand what is at stake. Where the child does not display an understanding of the obligation of confidence, parents may be freely told everything about the treatment. While some lawyers accept that there are three possible categories: (a) those mature enough to consent to treatment, (b) those insufficiently mature for this but nevertheless still mature enough to be entitled to confidentiality and, finally, (c) those entitled neither to confidentiality nor to consent to treatment, others believe that the ability to consent to treatment and right to confidentiality cannot be separated, so that there are only two categories.

Whichever view is correct, parents have no automatic right to know what is happening, and even if the view of the present authors that there are three categories is wrong, nurses may refuse to answer parents' questions if exceptional circumstances indicate that it is for the child's good to withhold the information. Where the child is not entitled to secrecy towards his parents, the obligation still exists on the nurse in respect of other people, and the consent of a parent should be obtained before any disclosure of confidential information.

What happens if parents and children disagree?

The most difficult circumstances to deal with probably arise when the child and his parents disagree. In the *Gillick* case, the House of

Lords considered that the right to take decisions passed from the parents to the child when the appropriate stage of maturity was reached. Thus, if the child has the capacity to consent to the care about which there is dispute, the child's own view must prevail. If he or she does not have this capacity, then the parents may take the decision, even against the wishes of the patient himself. However, their refusal to accept the child's views could be challenged by using wardship or care proceedings (see below) if their decision seems seriously inappropriate.

How do children get into local authority care?

Sometimes it is necessary to supplement or supersede parental care. Alternative care of this sort will usually mean the involvement of the local authority social services department. If long-term arrangements are required, this can lead to children being adopted. Where this happens, the child becomes part of the new family and the usual principles apply as outlined in the first half of this chapter. Before then, the social services may be closely involved, possibly assisting or supervising the child's parents or perhaps arranging for the child to be fostered or taken into a children's home. In such circumstances, it is necessary to appreciate the role of the social workers.

The detailed circumstances when a child will be taken into care are quite specific but, broadly speaking, it will happen when it can be shown that the way in which they are being looked after significantly fails to reach acceptable standards. This must usually be, to some extent, the fault of the parents. Children are not automatically taken into care, just because such circumstances exist. Taking a child into care is a drastic step, and less coercive ways to solve the problems will be examined before it is taken. The Children Act 1989 will simplify the grounds on which children can be compulsorily removed from their parents. At the time of writing, it is unclear when it will come into force.

Under the existing law, there are many different ways in which a child is taken into care. Sometimes a care order will be made by magistrates in the Juvenile Court. Sometimes a local authority can itself decide to take over legal responsibility for a child already voluntarily entrusted to them by the parents. Occasionally, a child will be placed in local authority care by a court dealing with custody disputes between parents, for example in a divorce case. In all, there are some eleven routes by which a child may enter local authority care, and the grounds on which it may occur vary for each one. Under the new reforms, it will always be a court that takes the decision and the whole process will be much simplified.

There is also an emergency procedure whereby a child can be taken into care for a short period while his needs are assessed and more information is gathered. This will often be used when it is suspected that a child is being seriously abused. A 'place of safety order' allows a child to be taken out of a family and kept in a safe place (including a hospital) for a period of 28 days. After the end of this period, the full process of taking a child into care must be carried out. Such an order must be made by a magistrate, but anyone may apply for one if they believe there is cause for concern. The usual course of action that a nurse who believes that a child is at risk would take is to call in the social services. The police also have the power to keep a child in a place of safety even without a court order.

What are the effects of a child being in care?

Because of the complexity of the existing law, there are slight differences in the position of a child depending on the route by which he was admitted to care. Essentially, however, a child who is in care has had his parents replaced by the local authority's social services department. This means that decisions relating to his upbringing will be taken by them rather than his parents. These will include decisions about medical treatment and nursing care. Some of this responsibility, so far as it relates to day-to-day matters, may be delegated to foster parents. It will be necessary to check who should be consulted about a particular child patient who is in care. In the case of a child who is a ward of court, it will be the court itself when serious matters are involved. Similarly, where the child is under local authority care, decisions with long-term significance should be referred to the social workers concerned. Minor issues will usually be resolved by those to whom responsibility for looking after the child has been delegated (that is, the foster parents).

The position of the child's 'natural' parents will also have changed. They will no longer be able to decide what happens to their child. Normally, they will be allowed access to see him, but this is not automatic. Where it is suspected that children have been abused by their parents, it may be necessary to keep them away completely. It is therefore necessary to discover the circumstances of each patient. If parents have not been given a right of access, they should only be allowed to see the child with the express permission of the social worker dealing with the case. There may be similar complications in cases where a child's parents have been divorced. The parent who does not look after the child (that is does not have 'custody') will still very often be given 'access' and will therefore be entitled to visit him in hospital. Sometimes, however, courts do not allow this if it proves detrimental to the child.

A parent who has been refused access will probably not be entitled to detailed information about the child's care. Thus the consent of the social worker, the child if mature enough to be deciding what happens, or the custodial parent as appropriate, should be sought before information is given. This can create confusion and bad feeling, as happened in Cleveland, in 1987, in cases of suspected child sexual abuse. Nurses found themselves looking after children, some of whom were allowed to see their parents when others were not. In some cases, they did not know whether they should allow parents in or not. The social services were criticised for failing to properly inform the nursing staff of the status of their patients. Nurses should call for clarification if they are unsure of the position.

CHAPTER 11

People with infectious diseases

People who carry or suffer from infectious diseases present special problems for the law. Normally it is possible to allow patients to preserve their individuality fully because the only people who may suffer from their ill-health are themselves (see Chapter 5). Where their condition is infectious, however, further considerations arise. There is then a public interest in preventing the spread of disease in the community. In addition, the health professionals involved with care may need to be protected. As with those whose mental state is unstable (see Chapter 7), the basic principles have to be adapted to meet these special conditions. This chapter discusses the legal provisions which seek to balance these sometimes competing interests against each other. It will consider:

- the circumstances in which the freedom of patients may be restricted in the interests of public health;
- the circumstances in which the patient's right to refuse treatment can be overridden to protect public health;
- the obligations of professionals to care for patients with infectious diseases;
- the special application of the principle of confidentiality to patients with infectious diseases.

Special attention will be paid during the course of the chapter to the impact of these principles on patients who are HIV/AIDS-positive.

What legal powers exist to restrict patients' freedom?

The law in this area is now set out in the Public Health (Control of Disease) Act 1984. That Act provides extensive powers to help control the spread of 'notifiable diseases'. These are defined in the Act as being cholera, plague, relapsing fever, smallpox and typhus. The Secretary of State can add further diseases to the list, and local authorities may also do so with his approval.

The extension of the Act to any particular disease can be

geographically restricted, so that only some areas of the country are covered, in terms of duration, so that temporary orders can be made, and also in relation to the parts of the Act that are to apply to any particular disease. In respect of HIV/AIDS, for example, some parts of the Act have been applied and one section has been modified, but the condition has not been made a full 'notifiable disease'. As local provision can be made, there is no fixed list of notifiable diseases. Nurses should check with their employers the full list locally applicable and should be informed by them of any changes. Figure 11.1 lists the diseases which the Secretary of State has added to the category of notifiable diseases on a national basis. The full details appear in The Public Health (Infectious Diseases) Regulations 1988.

Acute encephalitis	Mumps
Acute poliomyelitis	Rubella
Meningitis	Whooping cough
Meningococcal septicaemia	Malaria
Anthrax	Tetanus
Diphtheria	Yellow fever
Dysentery	Ophthalmia neonatorum
Paratyphoid fever	Rabies
Typhoid fever	Scarlet fever
Viral hepatitis	Tuberculosis
Leprosy	Viral haemorrhagic fever
Measles	

Figure 11.1   *Diseases that are notifiable under The Public Health (Infectious Diseases) Regulations 1988.*

When a condition is a notifiable disease, several rules come into play. First, the existence and details of patients with the disease must be reported to the local authority, including their name, sex and address. This obligation falls upon the doctors involved not the nurses. The local authority must then inform the District Health Authority. Where school children are concerned, the local authority may require head teachers to supply a complete list of all pupils in the school in order to assist monitoring the spread of the disease.

Secondly, the liberty of those who carry notifiable diseases is restricted by the existence of several criminal offences. Anyone who knows that they are suffering from a notifiable disease will commit an offence if they expose others to risks by being in a public place, or by allowing contaminated clothing or other effects to be passed on to others without disinfection. Persons suffering from notifiable diseases are forbidden to use public library books, transport or laundry services. Anyone who is caring for such a person, including nurses, will be guilty of an offence if they allow them to create a risk of infection in a public place. It is also an offence to continue working once you know that you are suffering from a notifiable disease. People may be ordered to stop working by the local authority, in which case compensation will be payable by that authority. There is also a power to order that a child be kept away from school.

The third category of rules concerns steps that the local authority is empowered to take by the Act to help prevent the spread of disease, although they need not take action unless they think it is appropriate. These powers can only be exercised with the permission of a magistrate, who is to check that it is really necessary to do so. The first allows compulsory testing of persons suspected of being carriers or sufferers of notifiable diseases and also of whole groups where there is reason to believe that one of their number is a carrier. The second power allows a person suffering from a notifiable disease to be forcibly removed to hospital. This power will be available when a magistrate is satisfied that proper precautions to prevent the spread of the disease either cannot or are not being taken, that the risk of spread is serious and that suitable hospital accommodation is available. Finally, an infected person who is in hospital may be detained there, provided that a magistrate is satisfied that they would not go to accommodation that would allow proper precautions to be taken to prevent them spreading the disease. Note that this is phrased in terms of the suitability of the premises to allow precautions to be taken, not as an issue about the likelihood of the persons cooperating.

Special provision has also been made in relation to the death of persons with notifiable diseases. Bodies should be isolated, they should not be allowed to leave hospitals except for direct transfer to a mortuary or for immediate burial or cremation. Local authorities have a statutory duty to ensure quick disposal.

It is clear, therefore, that considerable inroads into people's autonomy and privacy are allowed in the interests of public health. Their right to refuse to agree to being tested can be overridden. Their freedom to refuse to go to hospital and to discharge themselves can be restricted. Their right to go where they please is limited. There is, however, no right under the statute to treat people against their wishes. The existence of the possibility of detaining patients until they are no longer infectious will be a powerful incentive to accept treatment, but it may not be forced upon them.

How far have these rules been extended to patients with HIV/AIDS?

HIV/AIDS is not a notifiable disease. However, some of the provisions of the Public Health Act have been extended to the condition. These provisions are those allowing compulsory testing of individuals (but not groups), the removal of a person to hospital and detention in hospital. The latter provision has been amended so that patients who are unlikely to take precautions can be detained, even though it would be possible for them to take them. These are all provisions that require the permission of a magistrate before the powers can be exercised. This is designed to prevent HIV/AIDS sufferers from being the victims of panic measures, although it is questionable whether it is a sufficient safeguard. The provisions dealing with the isolation of corpses have also been extended to HIV/AIDS, although not those dealing with disposal.

The AIDS (Control) Act 1987 requires health authorities to compile and submit to the Secretary of State reports indicating the numbers of patients with AIDS in their districts, and also detailing steps being taken to provide for testing, counselling and treatment of those with HIV/AIDS. Unlike those made under the provisions dealing with notifiable diseases, these reports do not contain information capable of identifying the infected persons. The problems of confidentiality, as they affect the responsibilities of nurses, are discussed below.

Can people be tested for HIV/AIDS without their consent?

The Public Health Act 1984 allows a magistrate to order people to allow themselves to be examined. As yet this provision does not seem to have been widely used. There has been much discussion, however, as to whether patients can be tested without their knowledge. This is usually proposed either as a protective measure for health professionals, or as justified in the public interest as part of the collection of information about the spread of the disease. As yet, the law has not been required to set down the principles that govern testing without consent, but it is possible to consider what guidance is implicit in the general rules discussed in Chapter 5.

The overriding principle is that no physical intervention is permissible without the patient's consent. That consent will be 'real' only if the patient is given a brief explanation about the nature of the procedure involved and is not deliberately deceived by that explanation. It would, therefore, be unlawful to take someone's blood in order to test it for HIV/AIDS while telling them that it was for some quite different purpose. Greater difficulties arise where patients consent to giving blood in order for tests to be undertaken, but are not told that one test will be for HIV/AIDS. Here it might be argued that extra consent to the latter test is unnecessary because it is included in the general consent to being tested. It is unclear whether the courts would accept this argument.

They might draw a distinction between cases where the purpose of the test is to allow proper treatment of the patient and where it is to protect the interests of the public health or the professionals who are delivering care. In the former case, it is probable that the implied consent argument would be acceptable so long as no specific question about HIV/AIDS was asked by the person to be tested. In the latter cases, it is probable that the courts would require explicit consent to be given. This would be because an analogy with research would be drawn where it is generally assumed that, as the procedures are not intended to benefit the research subjects themselves, it is necessary to explain what will happen far more fully than is usually the case with treatment or care. If this is right then testing without consent to protect health care professionals will hardly ever be permissible.

Another argument has been made that testing for HIV/AIDS would not require consent at all because it came within one of the exceptional categories of procedures for which no consent is necessary. This is said to be because the physical intrusion involved is so minor as to be acceptable in the course of ordinary life. This is most plausible in cases where the only intrusion attributable to the HIV/AIDS test is the drawing of a little extra blood. The venepuncture itself would have been consented to because of the other tests to be performed. Even here, however, in view of the seriousness of the HIV/AIDS issue, it might be unwise to rely on the courts accepting this argument.

Therefore, the better view would seem to be that patients who are to be tested for HIV/AIDS should be asked to agree to the test being carried out. They are entitled to decline to know the result if they so desire. They certainly should not be tested if they have expressly forbidden the health professionals to do so. Nurses should therefore feel able to refuse to cooperate with secret testing on the ground that it may be unlawful. The RCN's adviser on HIV/AIDS has suggested that nurses should report doctors who perform secret tests. It may well be that the need to monitor the spread of the disease will be found to justify compulsory testing in some form, but it is unlikely that the courts could be persuaded that the law already allows this when the issue is so controversial. It is most likely that they will hold that it is a task for Parliament to decide whether or not compulsory testing should go ahead.

What special responsibilities do nurses have in respect of people with infectious diseases?

So far as the duties of a nurse to the patient are concerned, the general principles apply. Nursing those who might infect others gives rise to a duty on the part of nurses to take reasonable steps to prevent contagion. Where it is foreseeable that someone other than the patient might be at risk, the nurse will have a duty of care to them (see Chapter 3). Anyone who contracts a disease because a nurse was negligent in the way infection control was carried out would therefore be able to sue. This might include cases where patients are discharged too soon. Primary responsibility there will fall upon the doctor who discharges the patient, but a nurse who knew that the patient was still infectious and who failed to point this out to the doctor might be negligent.

Do nurses have any right to refuse to care for people with infectious diseases?

Nurses have no right to refuse to care for patients of whom they disapprove, or are afraid. To refuse to nurse a patient because he or she is HIV/AIDS-positive would probably be not only a breach of a nurse's contract of employment but also professional misconduct for which he or she might be reported to the UKCC. However, nurses are not obliged to put themselves at risk. It would be permissible, therefore, to refuse to nurse an infectious patient without the appropriate protective equipment. Consequently, nurses in accident and emergency units could legitimately demand proper gowns and gloves before risking infection with hepatitis B or HIV/AIDS through contact with blood products. It might well be that the courts would uphold a refusal to work with patients infected by a disease for which a vaccine is available until the employer provided the appropriate vaccination, but the courts have not yet had the opportunity to consider the matter.

Do nurses have any right to be compensated should they contract an infectious disease while at work?

Employers have an obligation to ensure that the workplace is safe (see Chapter 4). It follows that if a nurse contracts a disease that could have been avoided if proper precautions had been taken, then he or she could claim compensation from the employer. This will not give rise to claims in all cases where infection has occurred because it is necessary to show that the employers failed to perform their duties properly. Sometimes infection could not have been reasonably prevented at all. It is unclear exactly what precautions the courts will accept as reasonable. At the time of writing, a nurse is suing her health authority claiming that she is entitled to compensation for having contracted hepatitis B. She is arguing that the authority was in breach of its duty to protect her safety because they had not arranged for her to be immunised against the virus. It remains to be seen whether she succeeds.

Sometimes it may be possible to seek compensation from an individual who has negligently caused the transmission of the disease (see Chapter 3). This might be a fellow employee who failed to warn the victim that the patient for whom they were caring was infectious. If it is an employee's negligence that caused the contagion, the employer will then be vicariously liable to pay compensation (see Chapter 4). There is much debate about the possibility of suing infectious individuals who cause others to contract the disease through their carelessness. It is unclear when the law will allow such actions. A further difficulty may exist in the case of nurses claiming compensation for infection at work. It is probable that they would be held to be contributorily negligent if they failed to take appropriate precautions. The courts would expect them to know how to protect themselves.

In some cases patients may deliberately seek to infect nurses. For example, a patient may bite a nurse intending to cause contamination. This would constitute a criminal offence as well as a civil wrong. The nurse could therefore sue the patient for damages using the civil law. In this case, the action used would be battery not negligence and therefore no question of contributory negligence would arise. If the patient were to be prosecuted, then the court might order the patient to pay compensation. Even if this does not happen, a nurse injured by a criminal act could seek compensation from the Criminal Injuries Compensation Board, which gives financial relief to the victims of crimes.

Can nurses inform relatives or others that a patient is infectious?

The principles of confidentiality that were discussed in Chapter 5 were designed to protect the privacy of individuals and to encourage patients to reveal information to health professionals candidly because they can feel confident that it will be kept secret. Where patients are infectious, it is necessary to consider whether confidentiality can be breached in order to protect others. This requires asking whether such a breach can be justified under the exceptions to the basic principle of secrecy.

The first exception permits disclosure of confidential information when the patient has consented. The safest course will therefore always be to seek to persuade the patients to agree to those close to them being told about their condition. Where they refuse to agree to this it will be necessary to consider next whether disclosure can be justified on the basis that the patients' care requires others to know of their condition. This might justify telling relatives if the patient is to be cared for at home, because special precautions need to be taken when disinfecting bedlinen or clothes. If the patient's relatives could not be told about the possibility of infection then the patient would have to stay in hospital, therefore it is necessary for the care of the patient to tell them. It is important that the need to know must relate to the patient's care, it is insufficient that the relatives need to know for their own safety. If that is the justification, then it is not a question of the 'need to know', but the 'public interest' exception.

The public interest exception is difficult to apply because it is so generally phrased. It is certainly permissible to break the obligation of confidence in order to prevent a crime being committed. Consequently, it is lawful to warn someone whom the patients says they will deliberately infect with the disease as that would be a criminal assault. It may be sufficient that the patient is expected to be so careless in respect of their hygiene that they would infect those with whom they live. Here there might be a negligence claim (see above). It is not so clear that a civil wrong of this sort will come within the public interest exception, but where there is an identifiable person at risk it is likely that the courts would accept that a nurse would be justified in warning them. However, the courts will not accept that the public interest justifies revealing the fact that someone is infectious unless there is some specific danger. There must be more than the possibility of infection, there must be the likelihood of infection of specific persons.

It is also important that confidential information is revealed only to the right people. It may be legitimate to warn the sexual partner of a patient with HIV/AIDS of the risks, but it will not be lawful to reveal the fact that they have the virus to a newspaper. Wherever possible, disclosure should be avoided and nurses must carefully consider how best to minimise the need to disclose information. These are matters that have not yet come to court in this country and it is impossible to be confident exactly where the lines will be drawn. It is unlikely that nurses who act in good faith will fall foul of the law, providing that they start from the assumption that confidential information should remain confidential unless it is absolutely necessary to reveal it.

Further reading

The following publications deal with their respective fields of the law in greater detail and in a more technical manner than this book has done. They are recommended for those wishing to explore further as they are written for readerships that are not expected to be expert in the law.

P. F. C. Bayliss, *An Introduction to the Law Relating to the Health Care Professions* (Ravenswood, 1987).
M. Brazier, *Medicine, Patients and the Law* (Penguin, 1987).
B. Hoggett, *Mental Health Law*, 2nd edn (Sweet & Maxwell, 1984).
B. Hoggett, *Parents and Children*, 3rd edn (Sweet & Maxwell, 1987).
T. Ingman, *The English Legal Process*, 2nd edn (Blackstone Press, 1987).
R. H. Pyne, *Professional Discipline in Nursing* (Blackwell, 1981).

Glossary

Attorney. This is someone who has been given legal authority to exercise legal power on behalf of another. This is called giving them a 'power of attorney'. Usually powers of attorney automatically become invalid when the donor becomes mentally incompetent, but if properly created as 'enduring powers of attorney' they can continue even then (see Chapter 8).

Battery means touching someone without their consent. It is a form of trespass.

Care order. A care order suspends the rights of parents to care for their child and authorises a local authority to do so.

Civil law. Deals with the relationships between citizens. Breaches of the civil law can lead to orders for compensation but not imprisonment.

Common law. The law developed from decisions of judges given in past cases rather than set down in statutes (see Chapter 2).

Court of Protection. This is a special office of the High Court, which oversees the management of the property of people who have been found incapable, by reason of mental disorder, of managing it themselves (see Chapter 9).

Criminal law. This deals with the relationship between the state and its citizens, forbidding certain actions (which then become crimes). Breaches of the criminal law can be punished by fines or imprisonment.

Defamation. This is a false statement about another living person, which damages their reputation. Very generally, 'libel' is defamation in writing, 'slander' is oral defamation.

Duty of care. To have a 'duty of care' to someone in the law of negligence is to be obliged to take their interests into account. It does not necessarily require that you do what is best for that person, but you must give them proper consideration (see Chapter 3).

Euthanasia. The term means 'dying well' and refers to practices that allow those who are dying to do so in the way in which they choose. 'Active euthanasia' is where steps are taken to lead to death, such as administering a drug to cause the patient's death. 'Passive euthanasia' means allowing the patient to die instead of trying to keep them alive. Euthanasia can also be voluntary (where the patient chooses to die) or involuntary (where someone other than the patient decides that they should die). Euthanasia is not encouraged by English law but passive euthanasia may in some circumstances be lawful (see Chapter 5).

Necessity. Under the doctrine of necessity, the usual rules are suspended because they come into conflict with a more important principle. Thus, for example, the rule that you cannot treat a child without the consent of their parents is suspended in respect of life-saving treatment because saving the child's life is more important than respecting the wishes of parents. This doctrine is discussed in Chapter 5.

Negligence. This is used by lawyers in two different ways. First, it can mean an area of law that permits one person to sue another for compensation (short for 'the law of negligence'). Second, it can be used to indicate that behaviour has fallen below required standards. In this latter sense, the word is sometimes used in criminal and employment law as well as the civil law.

Place of safety order. This is a court order that allows a child to be removed from his or her current situation and taken to a place of safety. This could be a hospital or police station.

Precedent. English courts adopt the principle that, if a law is interpreted in one way in one case, it should be interpreted in the same way in other similar cases. This is called the doctrine of precedent, and previous cases are called precedents.

Receivership order. An order made, in the context of health care, by the Court of Protection when a patient is incapable of managing their property. It requires that the patient's property should be given to a receiver to manage on their behalf (see Chapter 8).

Recklessness. An act is committed recklessly if the actor foresaw the risk of some harm but, nevertheless, went ahead or did not think about the harm when a reasonable person would have realised there was an obvious risk.

Short procedure order. This is a more flexible and less expensive procedure than a receivership order, for use where someone is incapable, by reason of mental disorder, of managing their own property (see Chapter 8). Unlike a receivership order, it can only be used where the amount of property is small or easy to deal with.

Standard of care. Standard that the law requires to be reached to avoid negligence.

Statute. This is a synonym for Act of Parliament.

Statute law. Statute law includes Acts of Parliament, regulations and statutory instruments made by government ministers. It contrasts with common law, which is 'judge-made' law (see Chapter 2).

Statutory instruments. This is a form of law-making by government ministers under powers given to them by an Act of Parliament. They are not usually discussed by Parliament, although they are made available to MPs for consideration before coming into force (see Chapter 2). They are sometimes referred to as delegated legislation.

Tort. A word used to cover the area of civil law, including negligence, trespass and defamation, which gives people rights against each other.

Trespass. This is the name given to the civil wrong (or 'tort') of touching or threatening to touch people without their consent or some other legal authority (see Chapter 5). It is divided into two categories. Actually touching is called 'battery', threatening to touch is called 'assault'. There can also be trespass to property.

Trust. This is where one person (or group of people) formally owns property, but does so on behalf of another. The person owning the property is called a trustee, the person (or people) for whom it is owned is called a beneficiary.

Vicarious liability. This is where employers are made responsible for the torts or civil wrongs (and sometimes crimes) of their employees.

Wardship. This is where a child (a person under 18 years) is put into the care of the High Court. They are then called a ward of court and no important step in their life can be taken without the court's permission. This can be used to prevent parents making decisions that threaten the child's future.

Index